Not Done Yet

For Joyce
with so much
thanks & with
love,
Laurie xox.

Not Done Yet

Living through Breast Cancer

Laurie Kingston

Women's Press
Toronto

Not Done Yet
By Laurie Kingston
First published in 2009 by **Women's Press, an imprint of Canadian Scholars' Press Inc.**
180 Bloor Street West, Suite 801
Toronto, Ontario
M5S 2V6

www.womenspress.ca

Canadian Scholars' Press Inc./Women's Press gratefully acknowledges financial support
for our publishing activities from the Ontario Arts Council, the Canada Council for the
Arts, the Government of Canada through the Book Publishing Industry Development
Program (BPIDP) and the Government of Ontario through the Ontario Book Publishing
Tax Credit Program.

Library and Archives Canada Cataloguing in Publication

Kingston, Laurie
    Not done yet : living through breast cancer / Laurie Kingston.

ISBN 978-0-88961-469-7

    1. Kingston, Laurie. 2. Breast—Cancer—Patients—
Ontario—Biography. I. Title.

RC280.B8K565 2009   362.196'994490092   C2009-900246-9

09 10 11 12 13   5 4 3 2 1

Printed and bound in Canada by Marquis Book Printing Inc.
Book Design by Em Dash Design

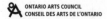 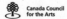

This book is dedicated to Tim, Sacha, and Daniel, who know me best and love me anyway.

Table of Contents

Introduction

THE MEMORY REMAINS A VIVID ONE. I was getting ready for bed on a Friday night, and as I undressed, my hand brushed against my right breast. I felt a large, hard lump.

At that particular point in my life, I was enormously busy. I was very much engaged with my work, doing research and communications for a public sector union. I was very ambitious and at a stage in my career when some great opportunities were about to come my way. I also had two young kids. I felt very conflicted by the pull between these two spheres of my life.

It had never occurred to me, except fleetingly (despite the fact that several women I worked with had been diagnosed in recent years), that I would find my life radically changed by breast cancer. And yet, at thirty-eight years old, that is exactly what happened.

The days and weeks that followed my discovery of the lump were spent wavering between panic and denial as I waited to confirm what I already knew to be true. I continued to work, welcoming the distraction of meetings and project management, but felt like I was outside myself, watching and thinking: *How can any of this matter when I probably have breast cancer?*

Some time during my last week of work (I went on leave a week before my scheduled surgery date), I sent out an email to my closest co-workers, advising them that I had cancer and thanking them for their friendship and support. I also informed them, as well as my friends and family, that they could keep up with my news and follow my progress on my blog, "Not Just about Cancer."

I didn't really read blogs before I decided to write one of my own. I was made aware of blogging through Tim, my spouse, who, it must be said, has been my steadiest and most enthusiastic supporter throughout the blogging process and indeed through my adult life, and who occasionally sent me links to blogs he thought I might find interesting. He helped me choose a user-friendly platform and carefully vetted my first, painstaking entries. To this day, he has never left a comment on the blog, but he has read every entry and almost always proofs my posts before they go "live."

Writing is something I have always done, even as a child, and I knew that blogging would provide me with a way to keep in touch with friends, process my own feelings, and perhaps reach out to others in the same situation.

I also knew that writing would help me remain in control of the flow of information that would result from my diagnosis and the messages that folks would be hearing. I thought it might give me some distance from my own feelings—by writing an online journal, I could hold them up and examine them, shape them, and keep them at a distance. This last point was the only part of my plan that did not go as expected.

I started the blog on January 12, 2006, and have been writing ever since. From the beginning, I found myself writing very openly, expressing things that I was not able to say out loud, and it did help me to communicate, work things through, and control how my story was interpreted. However, instead of distancing myself from my emotions, writing the blog helped me to embrace them. Expressing my doubts and my fears helped me get past some of the anger and the shame. As a result, I think I'm a much happier person.

At first, I wrote haltingly, rereading each sentence three or four times. Soon, though, the words started to flow more quickly. Sometimes I surprised myself by what I wrote. I documented doctors' appointments, surgery, chemotherapy, and the reactions of friends and family to my cancer. I wrote about my kids, my life, and people I met on the street—the blog is called "Not Just about Cancer" for a reason! I wrote throughout my triumphant return to work and the realization three weeks later that my cancer had spread to my liver. I even wrote a love letter to my blog after a hospital stay had kept me off-line for a few days.

As I wrote, I was embraced by a vibrant, caring online community. I began to receive comments, emails, and, on several occasions, gift certificates and packages in the mail. I became aware that my blog connected me to so many different people. Some I know in real life and some I may never meet in person. Many are folks like me whose lives have been affected by cancer. Others found something in my writing to which they could relate. I am still amazed at the community of interesting, progressive, talented bloggers out there (many of whom are very different from me on the surface) whose blogs I follow and with whom I feel an important connection.

I have been most affected by the community of strong, smart women who write openly and with great humour about breast cancer. Many are activists who, like me, are uneasy with the breast cancer industry and the profits it generates. And many, myself included, have found the urge to create, photograph, write, knit, or just generally "make stuff" to be a celebratory and even rebellious act in the face of cancer.

Shaping the blog entries into a book was much harder than I anticipated. It was very difficult to reread some of my posts, especially the earliest ones, and not relive the fear and the pain. Even the most joyful posts can feel bittersweet as I now know that the initial course of treatment would prove to be unsuccessful and that the cancer would return.

As I was trawling old blog-related emails, I found the following email I sent to a friend, shortly after my surgery:

> My life is going to be so very different for the next year than I thought it would be. Even recovering from surgery and accepting the physical limitations, the ugly scar, the fluid buildup, the pain.... It's just unbelievable that at thirty-eight, and the fittest I have been in my life ... well, suffice it to say that I am having tremendous difficulty reconciling how I usually think of myself with now being someone who has breast cancer.

I now know that I will always be a cancer patient, but that means something different to me than it once did, and the cancer itself and the process of writing about it have exposed me to facets of myself that I didn't know existed.

I will never, as I wrote in the blog, say that cancer is a gift, but my life as a cancer patient has been full of many wonderful opportunities and simple, joyful experiences as well as some very tough times. I am grateful to be able to write about it.

And I am very grateful for the privilege of being able to share my story again in these pages.

Part One

I Didn't Plan on This: Breast
Cancer at Thirty-eight

A Whole New World

Well, I've finally found a reason to create my own blog.

I am thirty-eight years old, have two young kids, and breast cancer. Since there has never, as far as I know, been anyone with breast cancer in my family, the odds of it happening to me are quite small indeed. Nor do I have very many of the other risk factors, but here I am.

I would rather have won the lottery.

I have, however, decided to deal with this challenge in the way I always do—along with liberal amounts of wine, outings with my dogs, and the abundant support of friends and family—by writing about it.

I have certainly found the experience thus far—from lump to diagnosis—to be interesting, or at least I have lots to say about it. And I hope this process will help me understand and explain this new world that has opened up to me.

What (Not) to Say

It's not easy to know how to respond when someone tells you she has breast cancer, but for goodness sake, say something. As hard as it is, and as awkward as you might feel, it is worse to say nothing than to mutter a few heartfelt words.

I'm not sitting in judgment here. I have missed several opportunities in the past to speak up when people I care about have been in difficulty. It feels so hard to find the right words. Trust me, though, if you don't acknowledge the elephant at the table, it just gets bigger.

"I'm sorry" is a perfectly acceptable thing to say. So is "That really sucks."

Some of the most meaningful things people have said to me:

"This is a campaign and we're going to win it."

"If I know anyone strong enough to deal with this, it's you."

"I know your treatment will be successful. You're a tough customer."

From a breast cancer survivor: "The majority of us will live long enough to die of something else."

Some more dos and don'ts:

* Do offer to help—if you mean it and you can.

* If you want to tell me a story about your friend/cousin/neighbour who had breast cancer, think ahead for a second. How does the story end? Unless your friend is now healthy and cancer-free, I don't want to hear it.

- Do ask me how I am, but don't act dubious if I say that I'm fine. At that particular moment, I might be, or I might just be trying really hard to keep it together. Either way, let me take the lead on whether or not I want to pour out my heart.

A word about God: I'm quite happy to hear that you are including me in your prayers. I'll take all the good thoughts I can, in whatever form. Don't, however, tell me that this is all part of God's plan for me because if I believed in God and thought he planned this for me, I'd be pretty pissed off at him right about now.

My Timeline: From Lump to Diagnosis with One Noteworthy Detour

December 2: *The Lump*

While getting undressed at night, I find a lump in my right breast. It feels about the size of a walnut.

December 3: *The Referral*

The next day is a Saturday, but I still get in to see a family physician. A very nice doctor, who looks about the same age as Doogie Howser was in that television series, is concerned enough to refer me for a mammogram.

December 8: *The Mammogram (and Ultrasound)*

After calling around, I am able to schedule a mammogram in less than a week. The mammogram itself, which involves having your breast mushed between glass plates, is no big deal—uncomfortable, but not painful. I had been told to expect my results within a week, but the technician comes back from developing my films looking very serious. She decided to show them to the radiologist on call, who referred me for an immediate ultrasound. Everyone I deal with from that point on looks very grim to me.

After the ultrasound, I am herded into a consultation room for an impromptu meeting with the radiologist. I don't remember much from this conversation except "It doesn't look good," and "Hope and pray for the best, but prepare for the worst." I also remember the word "urgent" being used several times. I later learned that this radiologist also called my GP to reinforce the "urgency" of my situation.

I do what any sensible person would do and spend the rest of the day drinking with friends.

December 20: *The Detour*

I'm on my way out the door when my doctor calls. She sounds furious. Instead of being forwarded to the cancer centre, my mammogram films are in the film library at the hospital. My "urgent" films have been put into storage. I drop everything, go pick up my films, and deliver them to the cancer clinic.

I receive a call the next day to set my biopsy appointment for early in the new year. I remember nothing from the holidays that year, except my determination to give my children as normal a holiday season as possible.

December 30: *The Second Lump*

I find a lump under my arm, about the size of a large raisin, or a small grape. This is new. It was definitely not there when my GP examined me on December 14.

January 3: *The Biopsy*

I have an ultrasound-guided biopsy of both lumps. Once I am injected full of novocaine, I feel nothing. I will be a little sore for the next couple of days, but all in all, I am more traumatized by the sound the larger needle makes as it takes the sample from my breast (a loud sort of *kachung!*) than by physical discomfort. Also, I'm not really sure why, but I am unable to raise my arm above my waist for the next twenty-four hours.

January 5: *The Diagnosis*

My GP calls me at work with the news I have been expecting, but still hoped not to hear. I have cancer. Technically speaking, I have "infiltrating ductal carcinoma in my breast and metastatic adeno-carcinoma in my axilla that is consistent with the carcinoma in the breast." (Translation: Garden variety breast cancer located in a milk duct. This same cancer has spread to my lymph nodes.)

January 13: *The Surgeon*
My surgeon is quite small physically, but the size of his ego more than makes up for his lack of stature. The good news is that my physical exam reveals no lumps above the collarbone—this is a huge relief. The not-so-good news is that my tumour appears to have grown to about 5 cm, the size of a plum, to continue using fruit as comparators. My surgery will take place February 2.

Three observations:

1. I must act as my own advocate. I'm not sure that the snafu with my mammogram films would have been discovered so quickly if I hadn't been pestering my GP and the cancer clinic with daily phone calls. As a cancer survivor put it to me, "People may be concerned and mean well, but it's your life that's at stake."

2. Our public health care system does work reasonably quickly and well, and the competent, caring health care practitioners have, in my experience so far, been the rule, not the exception. Let's see if I still feel this way in a few months' time.

3. One should always bring a small army of supporters (or at least one very good friend) to every appointment.

Getting to the Root of the Problem

Modified radical mastectomy.

I couldn't say these words for three days without my voice breaking. It's taken me more than a week to be ready to write about it.

My surgeon is compassionate, yet blunt. After examining me, he told me that my tumour is too "bulky" to do a lumpectomy. His exact words were, "It would look like hell."

He also asked me how I would feel if he told me he was going to take out "only some of the cancer." Not that I was arguing. I was shocked and silent, my brain trying to catch up with all the information that was being thrown at me.

The surgeon did offer me neoadjuvant chemotherapy—chemotherapy given before surgery in an attempt to shrink the tumour so that a lumpectomy (or breast-conserving surgery) can be performed. He said that studies in the US have shown this process to be successful 65 percent of the time. In his personal experience, results have not been so good and women have often still needed to have the mastectomy.

The surgeon said I could take some time to think about it if I wanted, but I could tell which way he was leaning, and while he does seem to have a bit of a God complex, he is also very confident and has an excellent reputation, so I signed the release form. And then I went home and fell into a deep funk.

I have always had an ambivalent relationship with my breasts. They have been a source of pride and shame (I am both a product of Western culture and my Catholic upbringing). They have fed two children for a total of forty months. When I weaned my boys, I felt both sadness and relief. Only recently have I come to feel comfortable in my own skin, to like what I see in the mirror, this familiar body.

And now it will change, dramatically and permanently.

Modified. Radical. Mastectomy.

I'm assuming that those who read this will know what a mastectomy is.

The modified part means the surgeon will also do an axillary dissection, the removal of my lymph nodes.

And radical means "root," as in getting to the root of the problem—hey, I learned something in university! And this is what the surgeon and I are choosing to do. I have come to terms with my decision. It is the right choice for me. At least I feel that way most of the time.

Before he wrote my name in his calendar beside February 2 ("Groundhog Day!" I exclaimed; I then had to explain that I wasn't objecting to surgery on Groundhog Day), my surgeon said, "I will cure you."

I went for a run with one of my two dogs in the snow today. It was hard work, but breathtakingly beautiful. And the joy of a dog in the fresh snow is contagious.

I'm writing this while sitting by my small son's bed. He's pretending to be asleep.

Right now, at this moment, it feels easy to be hopeful.

■ **Monday, January 30, 2006**

Being (a) Patient

There is nothing like sitting in a cold waiting room wearing an unflattering robe and your winter boots to test both your patience and your dignity.

The latter part of the week that just ended was filled with a gruelling round of preoperative appointments:

Wednesday, January 25

Location: The hospital where my surgery will take place

Admitting: I am issued with a green plastic card with my name, address, etc.

The pre-op nurse: A nurse fills me in on the details of my upcoming surgery, what I need to do to prepare, and how to follow up. She is very calm and thorough, and I remember almost nothing that she said to me. I am grateful for the written material they give me and for my friend taking notes.

The physiotherapist: I am provided with exercises to regain flexibility and strength in my right arm after surgery (and to ward off lymphedema, painful swelling in the arm that can occur as a result of the removal of the lymph nodes). I am expected to start these exercises the day after surgery and to progress gradually until I have recovered fully. I find this appointment very reassuring.

The home care nurse: I remember two things from my meeting with the coordinator of the home care program:

1. A nurse will visit me after the surgery and at least one other time after that.

2. The reply to one of my questions: "Oh, you should talk to the pre-op nurse. She handles all of Dr. M's breasts." I refrain from pointing out that I still think of them as my breasts, despite the fact that Dr. M. will be removing one of them.

Thursday, January 26

Location: Different hospital, nuclear medicine

The bone scan: I had been told to arrive at 8:15 in the morning, when I would be given a drink to prepare for my bone scan later that morning. Instead, I am injected with "a small amount of radioactive material" and told to return in two hours.

After cooling my heels for a while, I am ready to be scanned. This process involves lying on my back while a camera passes slowly over me. The five minutes spent with the camera directly over my face (not touching but really, really close) are a bit weird, but otherwise the process is painless.

My oldest son is really impressed with the idea that I have been injected with radioactive material. We conduct a series of experiments and prove that, unlike Spiderman, the experience has not given me superpowers. I don't mind. Those superheroes lead pretty lonely lives.

My friend and I notice a sign in the waiting room: "Please notify us if you are preparing to travel by air in the near future and we will provide you with appropriate documentation." Apparently the stuff with which I have been injected can set off airport security alarms. Scary.

Friday, January 27

Location: A publicly funded private clinic

The abdominal ultrasound: The attire *du jour* is a white paper poncho, open at the sides and tied with a blue ribbon. It looks particularly fetching paired with my black Blundstone boots.

The technician is motherly (actually uses the phrase, "atta girl!"), and like all the others, is very nice. She has me breathe in and hold the breath more times than I can count. I forget to breathe out at one point as it suddenly occurs to me that although these tests are routine, they are meant to determine if the cancer has spread beyond my lymph nodes and into my bones or internal organs.

The chest X-ray: A run-of-the-mill X-ray, with front and side views. This is the first technician to mention the fact that I have breast cancer.

The heart scan (aborted): I was told by the woman at the cancer centre who had booked my appointments that this last step would be further blood tests. I am, therefore, a little surprised to be taken through a door with a now familiar graphic and the words "nuclear medicine."

After being seated in a tiny room, identical to the one I'd been in prior to my bone scan, I have the following conversation:

TECHNICIAN: "Are you ready for this?"

ME: "I don't know what *this* is."

TECHNICIAN: "We need to scan your heart to make sure that it's strong enough to withstand chemotherapy."

ME: "Is it really safe to be injected with radioactive material two days in a row? I just had a bone scan done yesterday."

TECHNICIAN: (Silence)

She then goes off to check with the doctor and, after a short wait, I find myself once again under a camera. The doctor (to whom I am never introduced) comes in, and after a brief, muttered conversation, I am informed that my ribs and sternum are still "glowing." A heart scan will be impossible.

This may seem like no big deal, but I had really been counting on having three whole days with no appointments prior to my surgery. Now half of Monday will be lost to more waiting rooms and another test.

I am told that it would have been okay for my *heart* to still be radioactive when my *bones* were scanned. If the two days had been reversed, I could have had my heart scanned, and then done the bone scan the next day. While this setback is minor, it is another example of how patients are right to ask questions when something that is communicated to us does not make sense. Even with the most skilled, compassionate staff involved in patient care, these breakdowns in communication seem to happen with a fair amount of frequency.

I had a two-hour massage today. It turned me into mush for the rest of the day, but did take the edge off my anxiety. I'm fortunate to have this kind of resource at my disposal, as well as family and friends who have overwhelmed me with their kindness and understanding. I'm also glad that I continue to see the humour in all of this.

Groundhog Day

Tomorrow is Groundhog Day. Thursday. The day of my surgery. I'm a little freaked out, but, I suppose, I'm as ready as I'll ever be.

I have been completely overwhelmed by the love and support people have shown me since my diagnosis. It has helped more than I have been able to express. If it weren't for my family and my friends (and the compassion of a few complete strangers), I would not be able to face what lies ahead.

I really wish I didn't have cancer (and I still can't quite believe that I do), but it has served to remind me how fortunate I am.

When I've recovered enough to type again, I'll write a little more about what I've been feeling and some big thoughts I've been thinking.

Right now, I need to have one last glass of wine and go turn my room into a proper nest. No doubt Mr. Groundhog would approve.

It Wasn't That Bad (or at Least Not as Bad as I Imagined It Would Be)

My father-in-law says that during his cancer treatment, he had to ask his spouse to stop being so nice to him—he was finding it disconcerting. His wife is a lovely woman and they seem to get along just fine, but I do take his point.

If food equals love, I am very loved indeed. My fridge, freezer, and cupboards are bulging with wonderful food, both healthy and decadent. Friends have brought me flowers, books, and a host of wonderful presents. I have been overwhelmed by this outpouring of support. And I'm enjoying every minute of it.

The hardest part was saying goodbye to my spouse in the waiting room, or rather several goodbyes before the nurse made him leave.

From then on, I was very well taken care of by everyone at the hospital—doctors, nurses, orderlies, volunteers. The hospital staff did everything they could to keep me warm and comfortable (heated blankets!). The surgeon came to see me to answer any final questions. He told me that he knew it was going to go well.

The last thing I remember after walking into the OR and climbing up on the table is a moment of sheer unadulterated terror (a nurse was arranging some very scary-looking surgical instruments) before the anaesthetist started asking about my kids and I relaxed and drifted off.

I woke up in the recovery room. I was thirsty and hungry and in pain. Water, crackers, and Demerol were administered in short order and I lay there for some hours, oblivious to the passage of time.

My surgeon came in to check on me at some point and delivered the news that the tumour in my breast had not affixed itself to my chest wall (good news in terms of cancer treatment and recovery from surgery, as it meant that Dr. M. did not need to cut into my chest muscles).

By 3:15, eight hours after arriving at the hospital, I was on my way home.

I never thought I'd say this, but I now understand why mastectomies are done as day surgery. I was in my own bed, able to see my kids. I felt safe and, well, "at home." I'm sure this contributed to my recovery.

A home care nurse came the night of my surgery (to administer another lovely shot of Demerol), the next day, and one last time yesterday to change my bandage. Since the first day, I have managed with Tylenol 2s for pain (and I'm no hero when it comes to pain management).

And here's the most surprising part: It doesn't even look that bad: One incision and a neat row of staples that will be removed in a week's time. That's the upside of imagining the worst. When I screwed up the courage to take a peek after surgery, I fully expected to see a bloody stump where my breast used to be. Instead, there was just a single narrow bandage that ran the breadth of my chest. And it's healing well.

Today I even went out for lunch, with a baggy jacket on. No prosthesis until the healing is a little further along.

Right now, the worst I have to contend with is swelling in the area where the lymph nodes were removed and in my upper arm. It can still be painful, but even that is getting better with time, elevation, and exercise.

My surgeon should call in the next day or two with my pathology report (grade, stage, and the results of tests for hormone receptivity). I assume that I will be meeting an oncologist shortly after that and in a few weeks' time, chemotherapy will start. I've already lined up a friend, who spent many years bald by choice, to shave my head before chemo does its worst.

When I admitted to struggling with letting people do all these things for me, another friend said, "We are grateful to you. When something like this happens, people feel powerless. Helping makes us feel less powerless." That helped a lot. People are doing for me and for themselves. That makes it easier to accept.

I really believe that if I am doing well, it's because of all the caregivers in my life, at the hospital, at home, and in my community. There are moments when this all seems too awful for words. My arm hurts, I'm exhausted, and scared, but it helps immeasurably to know that I am not going through this alone.

This is why I am also grateful to the friend who opened a phone conversation with, "Are you listing to one side?" Her girlfriend was appalled, but I couldn't stop laughing. That was a gift, too.

The Roller Coaster Takes a Downturn

It was bound to happen. I finally cried last night.

The English language is full of descriptive expressions that I have come to understand viscerally in the last couple of months: Heavy heart, heartbreaking, gut-wrenching, wracked with sobs. When the dam finally broke, I cried with my whole body until my chest ached and my throat was raw.

I was crying for how awful this is—being "sick," disfigurement, fear of dying, the prospect of chemotherapy, anger and fear that I can't and won't be there for my children, losing my hair, early menopause, all the horrible side effects of cancer and its treatment, losing myself as a sexual being, and how it's possible to feel loved and cared for and still be so utterly lonely.

It really was bound to happen at some point, and I guess it was good that it did.

Having cancer is really, really hard.

Moving Forward—Slowly

Call it hubris.

One should never post on the Internet how easy one's recovery has been from surgery when one does not really know what one is talking about. One definitely should not crow about it.

Within a day or two of my cathartic crying jag, I was on much more solid ground emotionally, but finding the fallout from surgery a little harder to handle. There was more pain, and a buildup of fluid at the site of the surgery that had to be drained twice. Scar tissue has developed under my arm and near my shoulder (my surgeon calls it a "web"; it looks more like rope to me) that should go away over time, but has greatly impeded mobility in my right arm.

Several people who've had surgery as adults have told me that this kind of backsliding is normal. I did find it discouraging, especially as I was trying to work last week in a context that was particularly stressful.

I do seem to be on the mend again.

I got my pathologist's report yesterday. My tumour is smaller than I had thought (4 cm) and had spread to four of the thirteen lymph nodes sampled. They also found another kind of cancer (ductal carcinoma in situ) in another part of my breast, but it does look like they got it all (the advantage of mastectomy over lumpectomy). The cancer was graded 3/3, which means that it is very aggressive. My surgeon says that is to be expected, given my youth, so ... good news and bad news as they say, but, generally speaking, things could be worse. My surgeon stages my cancer at a 2b (with stage 1 being small and with no nodes affected and stage 4 being cancer that has spread beyond the lymph nodes).

I am now on the waiting list to see an oncologist. Next step: chemotherapy.

I messed with my own head a bit last night by looking up the survival stats for those with my stage of breast cancer. I then reread a wonderful article by Stephen Jay Gould on cancer statistics called "The Median Isn't the Message." One thing the author writes about is the documented evidence that a positive attitude and belief in one's own survival contribute greatly to battling cancer successfully.

I should be fine.

A Boy in the Bath

My son Daniel lives in the moment. I am trying to learn from him.

Daniel is two or, as he says, "at my next birthday I be three." Tonight he had a bath. This is a small victory in our house. For months now, mere mention of bathing has been enough to make him run screaming from the room.

Tonight, he willingly climbed into the bath, washed himself, played with his toys, his fears forgotten. I had to pull the plug to get him out and even then he didn't notice until the tub was empty, inquiring, "Where did the water go?"

After we put his Spiderman pyjamas on ("Grammy gave these to me") and brushed his teeth with his Sponge Bob toothbrush (the influences of an older brother), he climbed into my lap for a story (poetry, actually—*Garbage Delight* by Dennis Lee).

I watched his face as he took in the pictures, completely absorbed. He belly-laughed at some of the silly-sounding words, and then he climbed into bed to read to himself. Daniel can focus completely on whatever is right in front of him, whether pleasure or irritant.

My older son, Sacha, is a dreamer and a worrier (at seven, he's a child who would lie awake worrying about cancer before he knew his mother had it). He finds it very hard to be in the moment, anticipating the next activity so much that the present goes by unnoticed. I am like that too. Sometimes it has served me well, helping me to plan and anticipate problems before they arise.

But both Sacha and I need to learn how to enjoy what is happening right now and not lose sight of that in anticipation of the future.

My children are growing up so quickly. Every age is interesting, challenging, and fun. They are so different from each other, but both are such beautiful, engaging, and interesting kids. I need to stop rushing ahead in time so I can enjoy them more, and savour each moment with them, especially now.

I have my first appointment with the oncologist on Monday, and then an appointment with a radiation oncologist a week after that. This is much sooner than I expected to hear. Good to move ahead, but also a little frightening.

I am going to try and enjoy this weekend—and every moment—to work very hard at not worrying about what the coming weeks will bring.

Chemotherapy (Part 1)

Today I learned that if I throw up on my clothes in the first forty-eight hours after receiving chemotherapy, I am to put them in a plastic bag and take them to the cancer centre, where they will burn them. I am not making that up. Chemotherapy is very scary stuff.

On March 9 and every third Thursday thereafter, I will spend at least three hours in the chemotherapy room, being infused with a toxic cocktail. I will do this six times. Then, after a break of a couple of weeks, I will be radiated every Monday to Friday for five weeks.

Being a cancer patient is a full-time job.

Chemotherapy (Part 2)

This is what it was like to get chemotherapy:

1. The Vampires

   They're actually three attractive nurses, but the women who work in pharmacology were introduced to me as the vampires, and I will always think of them as such. This is where I had blood drawn and ended up performing a duet of "Patricia the Stripper" (Chris de Burgh, circa my misspent youth), to which, I was astonished to realize, I remember all the words.

2. The Chemo Room

   This is a large room with a nursing station at the centre. At a guess, there are at least thirty of us receiving chemo around the room's perimeter at any given time.

   Before we begin the infusion, an oncology nurse goes over my extremely complicated post-chemo drug regimen. I have seven different prescriptions to be taken at varying intervals over the next several days.

3. Red Devil

   The first chemo drug is nicknamed this way by the oncology nurses because it's bright red, it burns, it's the one that guarantees hair loss, and you excrete bright red after it's infused. The "Red Devil" takes fifteen minutes to do its work.

4. Icy Fingers

   After an hour's break, during which I receive saline, it's time for the Taxotere, famous for the fact that it can make your fingernails turn black and fall out. In an attempt to prevent this, patients are encouraged to spend the hour and fifteen minutes of treatment with their gloved hands in ice. (I am reminded of my Pearson College economics prof: "A statistician is someone who has his head in the oven and his feet in a bucket of ice and says, on average, he's comfortable.")

5. The Closer

   The last drug is a walk in the park because I can move my arm and thus read. It takes about half an hour and then, after my vitals are taken, I am free to wobble off home. All told, I have been at the hospital for nearly six hours.

Tim, my spouse, has observed how surreal it is that an experience can be simultaneously so intense, yet so unbelievably boring. Thank god we brought music. Greg Brown, Jesse Winchester, Johnny Cash, and the incredible Melissa Etheridge got me through it, along with the aforementioned very patient spouse.

■ **Monday, March 20, 2006**

Going Bald

Last weekend (after the first round of chemo), I shaved my head. The wisdom of others (and my own gut) told me that even though I had very short hair, it would be infinitely easier to have it fall out in bristles than in thick clumps.

It turned into a bit of a party. Who knew so many people would want to watch me shave my head?

My friend Liam, who sports a tattoo under his now-conservative haircut, did the honours. I don't think he was expecting it to be a performance, but he took it all in stride. And he donated the clippers. What a guy.

We had a wonderful evening. And I think it's made the whole going bald thing much easier for my kids, as well as for me.

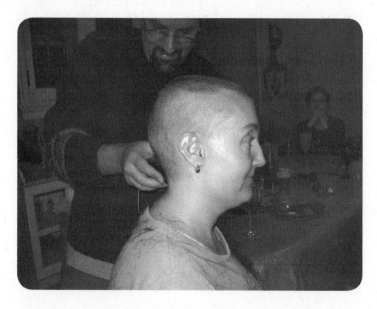

Thursday, March 30, 2006

Chemotherapy (Part 3: The Grim Aftermath)

Two down, four to go.

Feeling a little "off" after this morning's chemo, but okay. Anxious, though, because last time I was fine for the first twenty-four hours and then became very sick.

I spent the weekend curled up in the fetal position, in agony, unable to deal with sound, light, or movement. On the Saturday afternoon, I had the home care nurse come and give me an injection of an anti-nauseant, which helped me keep the oral medicine down.

As for eating, once I could keep food down, chicken soup and soda crackers were the only items on my menu. That's tonight's dinner.

Once the nausea subsided three days later, I started to experience the bone pain associated with the injection I get after each round of chemo to keep my blood cells up (at $3,000 an injection). I also had an unbelievable case of the jitters and restlessness (like I'd had three pots of coffee injected directly into my bloodstream) and a weird twitch in my hands (couldn't knit or type). I was beside myself. Turns out that was a side effect of one of the anti-nauseants, which I've now been told is also a powerful anti-psychotic.

We've tinkered with my drug regimen slightly this round and I'm going to acupuncture tomorrow. Hopefully that will help. This is all so surreal. I still can't quite believe I'm this person with cancer and have seven different prescriptions to take at bedtime.

On the other hand, when the fog lifts and the nausea subsides, I feel joyous (I have a friend who is going through this at the same time I am and she describes this feeling as euphoria). I feel so damn grateful not to be sick that everything seems wonderful. I have grabbed onto those days and carry them with me because I know they'll come again.

I've been listening to a lot of music lately. The album of choice today is *Casino* by Blue Rodeo, in particular the tracks "Till I Am Myself Again" and "What Am I Doing Here?"

Not very subtle, I know.

The Importance of Books

I can always tell that I am beginning to turn the corner after chemo when I'm once again able to read.

I have loved books and reading ever since I was a little girl. My sister and I were taught from an early age the value of reading and were encouraged to treat our books with great care.

They say that to turn a child into a reader, you must read to them and make books available. The single greatest factor, though, in terms of turning young children into life-long readers, is having parents who read themselves.

My father was always an avid reader. He still is. Books are pretty much the only presents he wants from his daughters for Christmas, and we go to great lengths to supply him with ones he will like.

I grew up in a small town that did not have any bookstores. It did, however, have a library, and some of my fondest childhood memories come from the hours I spent there. I worked my way pretty quickly through the library's children's books and I was still quite young when I was allowed an adult card, which granted me access to a whole new world of books and unlimited withdrawals. (I don't really remember how old I was, but I don't really remember learning to read either. It feels as though I always have.) I was so proud.

I would spend hours prowling the stacks, pulling books off the shelves indiscriminately. *Pride and Prejudice* (I read it for the first time when I was eight years old), *Born Free*, *The Grapes of Wrath* (I read it when I was eleven, at my father's recommendation), or a book on transcendental meditation. I didn't discriminate much. If a title, an image, or a blurb on a dust jacket captured my fancy, I would read.

I remember going to a bookstore in a shopping mall in suburban Montreal at the beginning of family vacations. My parents would let us choose an armload of books. To this day, I still get excited when I walk into a bookstore. My heart beats faster at the world of possibility. And I love the smell of new books.

Then, when I switched to English school in grade 6 (I attended a local French school from kindergarten until grade 5), I discovered Scholastic Book Clubs. I would bring home a little newsprint catalogue, fill it in, my parents would write a cheque (we never had a lot of money, but books were always a priority and I don't ever remember my parents saying "no" when it came to a book), and a few weeks later, a little pile of books would arrive at the school for me to take home. At the time, it seemed too good to be true. Now, living in a city with many bookstores, a great library, and opportunities to order online, I often groan when my children bring home the Scholastic catalogues. I love their excitement, but I don't love that Scholastic now sells plastic toys and games to promote books based on television shows. I usually buy something, but try to steer them toward books they will read more than once.

And so, throughout my childhood, I read voraciously.

I read to escape the crushing boredom of a long, hot summer.

I read to be transported to worlds I could only imagine.

I read to make my father proud.

I read to escape.

I read on my play dates with friends. I read with a flashlight after the lights were out. I read in my closet.

I read whatever I wanted, with few restrictions (the only censorship in my family involved Harlequin romances and comic books, so of course I read those furtively). I read with a freedom that did not exist in the rest of my life.

Now that I am an adult, having been on adventures, and having done many of the things I once dreamed about, I still love to read. It is still a way to escape, be inspired, and be transported away from the challenges I am facing.

Curling up with a good book still soothes and heals. And the hardest days are the ones during which I am too sick to read.

Many people have given me books about cancer and I know that I will read them all some day, but not now.

These days when I read, I am not a cancer patient. I am a reader, an adventurer, immersed in the stories I am reading. Books get me away from it all, take me out of myself. Right now, I am reading books by young writers. How do they manage to write with such skill and depth at such an age? I marvel at their talent and their apparent confidence. And I start to fantasize about one day joining their ranks.

I read books in settings far from my own, with characters very different from me and the people I know, yet their stories resonate.

I am reminded of my newly discovered online community. Good writing also brings bloggers together across difference, and I enjoy reading them, too.

Boob in a Box

I went into my room to get dressed yesterday morning and found my new prosthetic breast sitting on top of its box.

My boys had been playing "pirate treasure hunt," although I think it was really an excuse for soon-to-be-eight-year-old Sacha to look for hidden birthday presents. I surmise the box on my shelf had been too much for two curious boys to resist.

I immediately went to tell Tim. Should I talk to Sacha about his find? Did he think it would be more traumatic if I talked to him or should I just let it go? My spouse, who had his hands full baking a cake for my three-year-old's birthday, said in so many words that he didn't think it was a big deal and that, while I could talk to him about it, I really didn't need to worry.

So I decided to wait for the right moment. A couple of hours later, I had the following conversation with my older son:

"Did you take something of mine out of that box on my shelf this morning?"

"Yeah. It was a pinkish, squishy thing. What was that?"

"Um. Well, you know when I had my surgery, it left me flat on one side. This is to make me look the same on both sides."

"Cool!"

Pause.

"So it makes you look normal."

"Yeah."

"Cool."

End of conversation. Kids really do take most things in stride.

Joy

I am fundamentally a "the glass is half full" sort of person. It's not that I am always in a good mood (those closest to me would be sure to tell you otherwise). In fact, I have struggled with depression since my teens, and need to work hard at staying healthy. It's just that if there are two ways to look at a situation, I naturally gravitate to the most positive interpretation.

That's why I can say that during these months of chemotherapy, I feel well half the time.

A clear physical and emotional cycle has emerged after three rounds of chemo. The first couple of days afterwards I feel light-headed and queasy. By the weekend (every chemo is on Thursday), I go into the "trough," which lasts for several days. I feel pretty awful during this period, but the symptoms are better managed than during the first round. By early the next week, I emerge from the worst, but go into an emotional funk. Last week I spent several days exhausted and furious at how different my life is right now from what I expected it would be.

Then I turn the corner.

I went for a walk last Saturday, bubbling over with everything that is good with the world—the sunshine, my beautiful children, my dogs, my eyebrows (thinner, but still there).

I seem to get a week and a half of feeling better (the effects of chemo are cumulative, so I know that this period could get shorter, but I know it will come), during which I am positively euphoric.

I love my family, my neighbourhood. I have the best friends in the world. I am getting the best of medical care. I am happy. The fact that I can't find anything in my cluttered mess of a house only bothers me a tiny bit.

Chemotherapy is very hard and I really, really hate it. I am, however, very grateful for this opportunity to experience joy, and to be reminded that, really, I have a very good life.

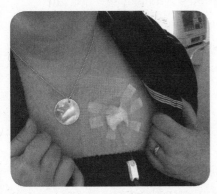

Strange Happenings

I love my job and when I'm feeling well, I miss it. It's hard not to feel some sadness and anger at times that life is going on without me, which, of course, it must. However, as my friend Cathy, who has been through this, commented the other day, this is a rare time in my life to be an observer, to really notice and think about life—the positive, the difficult, and the truly bizarre.

Listed below is a random list of some of the more absurd things I have observed and experienced in the last several weeks:

1. My insurance company requires a letter from my doctor detailing my diagnosis before they will reimburse me for my prosthesis (the prosthesis cost $350 and medicare pays for $180). "Why is this necessary? Who would buy a prosthetic breast just for fun?" I asked what I thought were rhetorical questions. Tim replied that it takes all kinds and that you never know what could turn up with a Google search. I don't dare try this.

2. My anatomy was recently enhanced with a portacath, a disk with some tubes attached that are connected directly to a vein that goes to my heart. It was inserted beneath the skin, a couple of inches under my collarbone, on my left side. It makes chemo infinitely easier as I can now use my arms during the hours I

am receiving treatment and no longer experience the burning sensation that I did when chemo was infused into a vein in my arm. Chemo also hardens and shrinks the veins, so the portacath is saving me the trauma of being poked repeatedly as the nurses try to find a vein in my arm. My portacath is a really nifty thing, but I do feel that I am more closely related to "the Borg" from *Star Trek* than I used to be.

3. Acupuncture is supposed to help with nausea, so I thought I would try it out. I've been seeing a doctor of traditional Chinese medicine who has considerable experience working with cancer patients. He also has a considerable number of eccentricities. For example, the first time I saw him, he greeted me warmly, then handed me a piece of paper stating that, as he suspected that someone was spying on him, he'd had a private security company in and they'd found listening devices all over his clinic (I have no idea if he is delusional or if this is true). Since that day, he asks that all his patients communicate with him in writing only—even while we are being treated. When he does talk, the doctor communicates chiefly in song titles: "You are always on my mind," and "I'll be waiting for you."

4. At my last appointment, my very cool oncologist suggested that smoking dope would be the best thing to alleviate nausea and other side effects from chemo. My mother-in-law responded by couriering me a pot cookie.

5. I took part in "Look Good Feel Better," a free session put on by the cosmetics industry. The idea is that women in treatment will feel better if they can be shown a few tricks to look more like themselves. And you get lots of free stuff (I love getting

free stuff). I thought it would be a lift, a bit of lighthearted fun, even if I left wearing more makeup than I usually apply in a month. However, the team leader for my session was a martinet, barking out orders like we were in boot camp: "Apply mascara now!" "Left hand on left eye! Right hand on right eye!" I spent the whole session frantically trying to catch up (and giggling madly).

However, when the martinet informed us that it was time for "a moment of silence to remember the fallen," I stopped laughing. I doubt there was a participant in that room who needed to be reminded of the "fallen." Or who hasn't had many moments of silence filled with the fear that we might join them.

Why I Write

I am not an exhibitionist. I think two or three times before sharing some of my more personal stories (for example, the decision to write about my mastectomy was not an easy one).

Writing for me has always been therapeutic, but that doesn't explain why I chose to expose myself so publicly.

I am doing this, in part, as way to keep friends and loved ones updated, as well as to help them better understand how I'm feeling and what this experience is like.

I am doing this because some aspects of cancer treatment are so strange that they must be shared.

I am doing this because our culture sometimes treats breast cancer like some kind of terrible secret, which in turn makes having cancer seem slightly shameful. Talking openly about my cancer makes people feel less awkward around me, which is much, much easier for me. I have always believed in acknowledging the elephant in the room, and while I respect the decision of others to keep their cancer a secret, it's really not the right choice for me. I guess I was pretty much an open book anyway (to mix my metaphors liberally) and don't see why cancer should change that.

A columnist in one of Canada's national newspapers recently scoffed at the idea of a cancer epidemic, talked about the cancer bandwagon, and said that of course there is more breast cancer now because there are more older people. She also dismissed the idea of environmental factors and the need for research into prevention.

I want that columnist and others who think like her to know that I'm here, thirty-eight years old, with no breast cancer in my family and very few of the risk factors associated with the disease. I really felt that my lump and subsequent diagnosis of breast cancer came from out of nowhere. I didn't choose to hop onto this particular bandwagon, nor did the many other women in my circle, including several diagnosed before the age of forty. I don't know if I would use the word "epidemic," but I do know that our numbers are growing and feel very strongly that the "why" of this must be further explored.

Finally, I am writing because, after my diagnosis, I found a dearth of stories about younger women with breast cancer and I thought that if I appreciate others' stories, then someone might like to read mine.

I Buy Myself Presents

It's true. Prior to each round of chemo, I have bought myself a present. I know that this is a really frivolous thing to do. I know that buying stuff won't buy me happiness. I also know that I am damn lucky to be able to afford such frivolity, thanks to public health care and a very good job with great benefits, but it really does make it easier to face the awfulness of chemo.

For the first round, I bought an iPod. This was a big-ticket item, but, in theory, the whole family shares it.

For the second round, I bought a teapot. I ordered it online as a replacement for one I had bought in London. I am pleased to say that it survived the flight over and arrived from England in one piece.

I bought two beautiful hats prior to round three from a local craft fair. They are both fine examples of millinery. Why two? Because I couldn't decide between them (please don't judge me). When I wore the black one (with a big green-and-red flower) to pick up my older son, he said, "You can't even tell that you're bald."

I have chemo this Thursday. On Monday I bought the most beautiful pair of red sandals. I had this idea in my head of a pair of very comfortable sandals for my longer walks, but with a bit of an edge. I found the perfect pair at the first place I looked. They are bright red. I wore them yesterday and two people stopped me on the street to ask where I had bought them. Joy.

Hot Flashes

They start in the morning, but come infrequently until the afternoon. By evening, they plague me in waves, starting up my chest, overwhelming me with heat until I am literally dripping sweat.

I almost took my clothes off at my son's birthday party two nights ago, thus ensuring years of therapy in his future.

I am experiencing what some call "faux menopause" or "chemo pause." The chemo has shut down my ovaries, my periods have stopped, and I am experiencing some spectacular hot flashes.

The night of my son's birthday (when, in my defence, I was under some stress), I became convinced that Tim was not being adequately sympathetic, that he just didn't get it, that in fact he was not being nearly supportive enough. And I told him so. Then I remembered that there are other menopausal symptoms. My poor spouse.

I have two friends who claim that their respective partners have offered to go out in the middle of the night, in the thick of snowstorms, to replace empty menopause-related prescriptions, such is the spousal fear of menopausal mood swings. My friends are both lovely women (and two of my heroes), yet they insist that this is true. Perhaps their spouses would like to form a support group with mine.

I know this is not the worst part of chemo—just insult to injury, really.

Fighting the Funk

Starting to resurface from the most recent round of chemo (no anti-nauseants today). Fighting the funk that seems inevitably to descend when I reach this place—basically, well enough to feel sorry for myself, but not to do much else.

To address this, I think it's time to make a list of things for which I feel grateful (not the big-picture stuff, but why, right now, today isn't so bad):

1. Sleep. I got much more of it this round.

2. My doctors and nurses ask about my side effects from chemo and seem eager to find the best ways to get through this. This has helped a lot (for example, no weird twitching this time).

3. I had just enough of my friend Bonnie's healing soup to get through the last few days. It was the only thing I wanted to eat this round.

4. While my dear old dog has a terrible sore on her leg, I have a vet who will come to my house to take care of her.

5. My house is clean, thanks to my mother, and I will not have to spend the whole time the vet is here feeling embarrassed.

6. I have only two more rounds of chemo to go.

7. I am able to write.

Another anecdote to add to my list of strange happenings: During a chemo session a round or two ago, I chatted a bit with the woman whose husband was in the bed beside mine. He has lung cancer and is taking part in a clinical trial involving infusing the patient with chlorophyll. The substance in the IV bag was definitely a very bright green. A couple of hours later, when the couple got up to leave, I noticed that the man was now green. He had not taken on a greenish tinge—he *was* green.

Another List

I need to make a somewhat random list of things I know about myself that have nothing to do with breast cancer:

1. I am the mother of the two most beautiful, sweetest, smartest boys to ever walk the face of the earth.

2. I am happily married to a real cutie, who will be both mortified and chuffed at being publicly called a "cutie." What the heck, he's extra cute when he's embarrassed. We have been together 15 years and we still make each other laugh.

3. I am crazy about dogs. I have two biggish beasties with sweet dispositions, who get me out in the world when I don't feel like going and who are the loveliest of companions.

4. I have put up for many years with a neurotic, malevolent tabby cat to whom I am unreasonably attached.

5. I knit. My knowledge and interest greatly outstrip my ability, but I love it.

6. Before the cancer, I had become a runner (albeit a very slow one) and I will be one again. Like knitting, I find it meditative and good for the soul, not to mention what it does for my legs. Also like knitting, running doesn't come naturally. It tickles me that two of the things I love best to do are things that do not come easily.

7. The first sign that I am starting to lose control over a fast-paced life: I lose things. It usually starts with my keys.

8. I have a somewhat addictive personality. When I get into something, it can become an obsession.

9. I am not someone who should own a BlackBerry (see above).

10. I love good coffee (black), good chocolate (dark), and good wine (usually red, but not always).

11. I love working in the labour movement and have a strong commitment to social justice. My spouse shares these values and I am proud to see my children absorbing them.

12. I have long been surrounded by a community of chosen family. Never have I been more grateful for this than in the last several months.

What I Need

It turns out that sometimes what I need to do is exactly the opposite of what I think I need.

Today, the only thing I wanted to do (and felt I could do) was stay in bed with a pillow covering my head, such was my fatigue and the blackness of my mood. I told my spouse this morning that I was "unfit for human consumption." I meant to say "unfit for human company," but my brain is in a chemo-induced muddle. However, the statement I did make is pretty accurate, given the toxicity of my chemotherapy regimen.

I had definitely been fighting a losing battle with the funk I have described in previous posts. I felt so overwhelmed by anxiety and despair last night and this morning that "just two more to go" had been wiped out by "I can't do two more."

I'm not sure why these first days when I start to improve physically are so much harder than the trough of the first few days after treatment. I know that impatience to feel better has something to do with it. Also, I get pretty stoned during much of the trough period, which is a good thing, so it is hard to muster up the energy to feel sorry for myself.

Then, when I regain a degree of physical energy, I am so happy to be out in the world that it becomes pretty easy to keep the dark thoughts at bay.

During these in-between days, though, it is a struggle not to dwell on the hard parts and the scary questions. How will I get through this? What if the cancer comes back? Why me?

Busy mind. Idle body. Bad combination.

And so my instinct this morning was to go up into the attic, never to emerge. Instead, I called a friend and had a vent and a laugh at the outrageousness of the world. I feel infinitely better.

It would seem that sometimes I just need to get out of my own head.

On another note, I just stumbled across a news release from Sunnybrook Hospital.* Apparently, women who over-express the protein HER2 (also called HER2/neu) benefit from more aggressive drug treatments (specifically the brutal "Red Devil," which I described in a previous post), while (and a whole host of other factors need to be taken into consideration) women who are HER2 negative may not. As someone who is HER2 positive, I found this oddly satisfying. I think it would have royally pissed me off (especially today) to find out near the end of treatment that I might have done as well on an easier regimen.

* Sunnybrook Health Sciences Centre news release, "Research Identifies Most Effective Chemotherapy Treatment for Premenopausal Women with HER2 Positive Breast Cancers" (May 17, 2006), www.virtualcancercentre.com.

■ **Sunday, May 21, 2006**

Chemo Brain ...

... is not just in my head. Finding the right word eludes me. Being consistently coherent is an unrealistic goal. My short-term memory is more or less non-existent. My brain has slowed right down. I've lost about a hundred consecutive Scrabble games. I really hope the damage isn't permanent.

"Don't Die"

We have an almost fourteen-year-old golden retriever who is nearing the end of her life. This dog has been my friend and companion through some very hard times and lots of good ones, and I will be heartbroken when she dies. So will my kids, especially Sacha, who is very attached to the old dog and who is himself old enough to understand loss and to fear death.

Sacha hasn't said anything to me about Emma-dog, but he talked to his grandmother about her on the weekend. He wanted to know how old his Grandma was, and was reassured to learn that, in dog years, she is still a spring chicken. He raised the subject again with Tim yesterday morning ("So, is Emma in the dying phase of life?").

We have all reassured Sacha that Emma is not suffering and that she has had a long and wonderful life. I think it's a very good sign that Sacha is working this through with us instead of keeping his questions and fears to himself.

Yesterday, before he left for school, he threw his arms around my neck and said, "Please don't die."

My mother-in-law and Tim were both with me when this happened and agreed that he was just fooling around, not realizing what he was saying until it was out of his mouth. I responded by laughing and telling him that I wasn't going anywhere.

But I wish I could protect my kids from having these thoughts, protect them from loss and death and fear. I guess all parents do. Instead, the best we can do is love unconditionally, listen when we are asked to, and let our kids know that it is as normal to fear and to grieve as it is to love.

Our dear old Emma may pass on soon and it will be very hard for my family. I want my kids to understand, though, that I am doing everything I can to make sure that I am around for a very long time.

In the Eye of the Beholder

My son Daniel is a supremely confident child. He goes through life secure in the knowledge that he is interesting, charming, and beautiful. People respond to him in kind. When he was a baby, I would often carry him in a backpack as I did errands. Every time, I would see even the most preoccupied strangers' faces break into smiles, reacting to my engaging child.

He is the centre of any group of children, regardless of age. Teenage friends of his caregiver's children greet us on the street and stop to shake his hand or ask for a hug. He is able to charm the dourest of adults and makes friends wherever he goes.

Daniel loves to play dress-up, picks out his own clothes, and cares whether his socks match his shirt, a concept that is foreign to his father and brother. One of his first sentences was, "I'm Daniel and I'm cute."

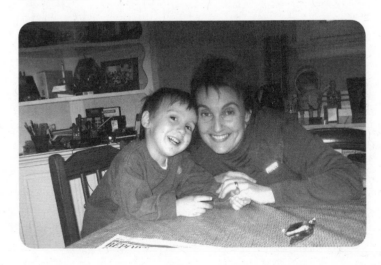

I have never, ever, thought of myself as beautiful, but Daniel looks a lot like me, and Daniel knows he is beautiful. And so, gradually, he has taught me to see myself as beautiful, too.

Now, I am bald and bloated. Surgery and chemo have taken their toll on my body, but if I look carefully, I can still see the beauty there. I have a nicely shaped head. There is still a sparkle in my eyes and warmth in my smile. I still have my dimple and the laugh lines around my eyes.

I may never enjoy dancing naked in front of our full-length mirror (one of Daniel's favourite pastimes). Daniel has taught me, however, that I have a choice in how I see myself.

I am still me. I am still beautiful.

Not Fair

Today's entry has been pre-empted by a bout of self-pity. Regular programming will no doubt resume shortly.

I am feeling pretty bitter today. I'm sick of being in treatment for cancer.

It's the National Capital Race Weekend and instead of running (albeit very slowly) in the half-marathon, I need to rest when I take my dog for a walk. It broke my heart to see the participants in the 10K stream down the street near my house today.

I miss my work and I am sick of feeling sidelined. None of my clothes fit me anymore. I am fed up with being stared at, even when the glances are sympathetic, but especially by those who are clearly uncomfortable with my appearance, perhaps because they don't want to believe it could happen to them.

I have lost patience with those who hurriedly change the subject when I acknowledge my cancer, as though I am being indiscreet. I hate looking and feeling like a cancer patient. I'm tired of handling other people's emotions about my breast cancer. I hate that my family is being made to live through this. I had a good life before my diagnosis (just six months ago) and I want it back.

■ **Sunday, May 28, 2006**

Better

The pity party is officially over. Life is too short to be spent wallowing and, besides, I have so much for which to be grateful.

I went for a long walk in the sun and had the chance to have fun with each of my children today.

I am exhausted tonight, but am feeling much more relaxed and content. I can get through this. In fact, I am a whole lot stronger than I thought I was before I knew I had cancer. This is something that will stay with me, I think, long after this struggle is over. What challenge could be tougher than this one?

I will get my life back. When I do, I will be ready for anything.

Of Fuzz and Fears

My hair is growing back. The patches that were completely bald (most of my head) now have a fine covering of fuzz. This makes me feel like I can truly begin to see the light at the end of the tunnel.

I had a second meeting with my radiation oncologist yesterday. He seems nice enough, other than being a bit paternalistic (I am increasingly irritated when medical practitioners speak to me as though I am a child) and also completely flummoxed by the fact that I don't have my husband's last name. ("But you are married to him? I suppose it's nothing personal.")

I'll start radiation two weeks to two months after I finish chemotherapy. Some women who undergo mastectomies are spared radiation. However, given the size and aggressiveness of my tumours, the oncologist believes that radiation could further reduce my chances of recurrence by as much as 10 percent, which doesn't sound like much, but every little bit helps, I guess.

Pros of radiation: Fewer side effects than chemotherapy and much shorter sessions (half an hour at most, compared to the three-plus hours of chemo).

Cons of getting zapped: Sessions are five days a week for five weeks; there is a likelihood of burns at the radiated sites, fatigue, and increased chance of lymphedema; no swimming (this matters only because I will likely be undergoing radiation during the hottest part of the summer); and the fact that radiation itself is potentially carcinogenic. I find this more than a little scary.

As we were leaving the hospital yesterday, I said to my spouse (only half-jokingly) that I thought I might skip radiation. It just seems like a lot of bother. Of course I'll do it, though. I need to feel like I have done everything I can to make sure the cancer never comes back.

Random Thoughts

There are trees in the cancer centre where I go to receive treatment—real ones. They built the building around them. They're a little spindly, but I love that they're there.

There is no rhyme or reason to what I want to eat after the first couple of post-chemo days have passed. This round it's shrimp soup, spaghetti, my spouse's super-high-fibre granola bars, and soda biscuits. The first couple of rounds it was chicken soup and pita. I think about food a lot these days and the pleasure I know I will get out of it when I turn the corner. My appetite tends to come back with a vengeance about ten days after chemo, and every round I have killed the time lying in bed imagining the things I am going to eat when I feel better. I also love that so many people have fed my family over the last several months. The impact of this food has been a source of sustenance that is much more than physical.

My cyclical funk has set in—too much time to think and too little energy to do anything or concentrate for very long. The lingering effects are relatively minor (mild nausea, light-headedness, a foul taste in my mouth, fatigue, and the surgical aches exacerbated by sitting still), but they serve as constant reminders that I have cancer. I did not fully expect how much of fighting this disease would be mental.

A poll of the medical staff at the cancer centre confirms that my new-grown fuzz will likely fall out again before chemo is done. It's okay. I have only one more round to go.

Bald Hypochondriac

I never see other bald women when I am out in public.

For the first several weeks of being bald, I kept my head covered in public all the time. Then it got hot, and I got sweaty, and the hat or scarf started to slide around on my head.

I just don't suffer in silence very well, so I've started taking off the head covering and offering up my head to the elements, or rather to the air conditioning. I do keep my head protected from the sun.

The first time I exposed myself like this, I was out at a nice restaurant with friends. I felt naked and acutely self-conscious at first, but became gradually more comfortable. My friend Bonnie remarked afterwards that there was at least one woman in the restaurant that night, hot and sweating in her wig, who was wishing she had the confidence to do what I had done.

I wonder if that's true. Given the cancer stats, there should be many more bald women out there. I'm not particularly brave, nor do I enjoy drawing attention to myself. I just don't have a high tolerance for discomfort. Am I violating some taboo I didn't know about? Where are all the bald women?

On another note, the depressed immune system from chemotherapy is exacerbating my not-so-latent hypochondriac tendencies.

My spouse took my youngest son to the doctor last week with a suspected eye infection, which I was sure he had given me. (Another child had been sent home from daycare with an infection earlier in the week and Daniel's eyes were suspiciously puffy.) All morning

I complained of itchy, watery eyes. I figured it was just a matter of hours until the infection would blind me completely.

I was stunned when my spouse called to say that Daniel did not have an eye infection. He had a mild case of tonsillitis. At least I can't become convinced that I have tonsillitis, too. I had my tonsils out when I was eight.

The Hardest Thing I've Ever Done

There is a sense of pride and accomplishment that comes with knowing that I have almost completed chemotherapy. Nothing I've ever done has been as hard as this. I am stronger than I thought I was. And tougher.

I know that I still have one more horrible chemo and the grind of radiation, not to mention Herceptin treatments every three weeks for a year, but I just realized today that the worst really is behind me.

Breast cancer has cost me a lot physically, mentally, and emotionally. I have not stopped being angry that it happened to me (and to other women in frightening numbers). I have, however, gained a sense of my own strength and the confidence of understanding what it means to be a survivor.

I know that others may have always seen me as confident, but I know how often I avoided challenges or situations that made me feel scared or intimidated. I think that will happen far less often in the future.

It's not that I don't expect to feel frightened or intimidated. It's that I know I can face those fears. I've written before that I did not anticipate how much of the fight against cancer is mental. I now know that I am brave enough to face a life-threatening illness and strong enough to survive treatment with my optimism and sense of humour intact. There are very few challenges that now seem insurmountable. That is the gift my cancer has given me.

Once More unto the Breach

Tomorrow is my last chemo.

I have not written much in the last few days because I have been too busy spending time with my kids and being hedonistic in my spare time.

I have spent my time with people who fill me up, who make me feel good about myself and fortunate to be in their presence.

I spent most of today with my friend Bonnie. We went for lunch, engaged in a little retail therapy (cancer presents: new clothes that fit my chemo-bloated body; I feel so much better about myself), and had a facial at the spa. When I told Bonnie last January that my biopsy had confirmed that I had cancer, she's the one who said, "This is a campaign and we are going to win it." Bonnie is a formidable woman. When she says things like this, I believe her.

On another note entirely, it turns out I am not as much of a hypochondriac as I thought I was. My oncologist took one look at me this morning and said, "Your eyes are irritated." It turns out that irritated, runny eyes are a common symptom of chemo, especially near the end. I feel vindicated.

For Emma Goldman Kingston (aka Golden Breeze Lady Emma Delight), b. July 17, 1992, d. June 29, 2006

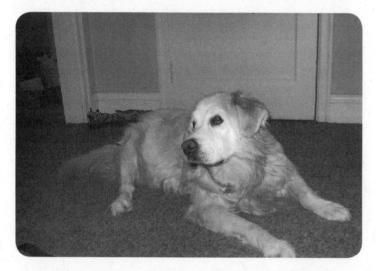

I am grieving an old and dear friend today. My dear old dog died peacefully in my arms this morning.

She had her head in my lap. We looked into each other's eyes. The first needle sent her to sleep. She began to snore gently.

After a couple of minutes, the vet said that it was time for the second needle, the one that would bring death. The snoring was silenced. The breathing stopped. "She's gone." I cried from the moment the vet arrived until after he took her away. I cried for Emma, at losing her, and out of regret. I cried because the last few months have been so hard and I have been so preoccupied. I cried because I felt guilty for feeling so relieved. I cried because all of this is so damned hard.

Emma, I love you very much and I will never forget you.

Sacha and I wrote the following eulogy together this afternoon:

We miss Emma because

1. She loved kids and always protected them, even when they didn't need protecting.

2. She was so affectionate with us.

3. She thought her name was "Beautiful Dog."

4. She enjoyed a good tummy rub.

5. She was the most stubborn dog we've ever met. From the time she was a round little puppy carrying tree branches, she did things her way.

6. She lived until she was almost fourteen and still loved us.

7. She once ate a dozen Chinese buns and was so full she could barely stand up.

8. There will never be another dog to replace Emma.

   And that's the truth.

What Passes for Normal

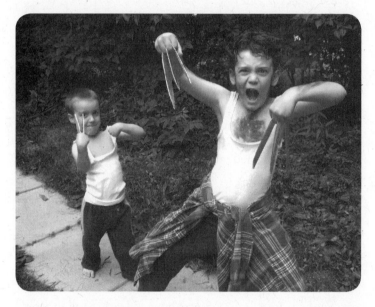

Today, the boys pretended to be Wolverine (as portrayed by Hugh Jackman in the X-men movies). They wore identical white under-shirts, but Sacha is the one who went all out, with a gelled pompadour and sideburns and chest hair (made from coffee grounds and petroleum jelly).

The boys were very pleased and we took lots of pictures.

We had a busy Canada Day with friends and family. I was feeling relaxed and quite celebratory. It slowly started to sink in on this beautiful long weekend that I am not recovering in order to get ready for the next round. I am done. No. More. Chemo. I am so relieved.

We are in chaos at the moment, trying to get organized to get out of town for a couple of weeks. The house is a mess, we are still working our way through our to-do list, and Tim and I have been more than a little irritable with each other. If we are all still speaking to each other, it will be good to get away. I'm going to pretend I'm not a cancer patient, just a very tired bald person.

I had my radiation planning session last week and am now in the queue for radiation. I could be waiting anywhere from two weeks to two months. I plan to use that time working at feeling healthy again.

Unfortunately, I seem to have developed lymphedema in my right arm, in addition to my chest and back. I am trying not to feel sorry for myself, but it does feel like the assault on my body has been relentless. I'm starting to wonder if I am ever going to catch a break.

Gobsmacked

Yesterday, I had the following conversation, in a cab, on my way home from seeing my shrink, a doctor I've seen a couple of times who works exclusively with patients who are recently bereaved or facing a life-threatening illness.

DRIVER: "How is life these days?"

ME: "Good, thanks."

DRIVER: "Are you a married lady?"

ME: (Don't ask why I answer these sorts of prying questions. It must be the first-born child in me, or the fact that I am stuck in this guy's cab with the doors locked.) "Yes."

DRIVER: "Your kids are out on their own then?"

ME: (See above) "No, they're not. They're three and eight."

DRIVER: "Oh! So it was a late marriage."

ME: "Not that late."

DRIVER: (Turning around to get a better look) "You look like you have no hair."

ME: (Sharply) "I have cancer."

DRIVER: (Chagrined) "Oh! I'm sorry." (Pause) "I shave my head most summers."

(Silence) "But I didn't this summer."

ME: (Politely) "Mmmm."

(Long, awkward silence.)

DRIVER: "So are you going to be okay? What do the doctors say?"

ME: "I hope so."

DRIVER: "Good, that's good."

I was enormously relieved when his cellphone rang. It was the longest cab ride of my life. Tim, when I told him the story, said, "Did you turn the cab around and go right back to the shrink?"

When given the choice, I prefer to laugh than cry. And a little righteous anger never hurt anyone.

The Wisdom to Know the Difference

I'm not much for prayer, but the first few lines of the "Serenity Prayer" are speaking to me today. I'm working on "the serenity to accept the things I cannot change" and "the courage to change the things I can."

I've been finding it hard to give myself the space to get better. I am tired of feeling like a cancer patient, and I want to feel like my old self again. I had a very important conversation with a very wise friend today about cutting myself some slack. She told me that it's not a failure on my part to admit that there are some things that I am just not ready to do. I really needed to hear that.

The pressure to have fully recovered is not coming from Tim or my family. It's something I'm doing to myself. I am impatient and I want to put treatment behind me. I also want to remind myself and others that I am smart and competent and that there is much more to who I am than cancer.

I read an interview with an oncologist yesterday who said that, in her experience, the time it takes to recover is the same length of time from the first sign of cancer (i.e., finding the lump) to the last day of treatment (not including Tamoxifen or Herceptin). If this applies to me, and radiation ends on September 6, I should feel like myself again in May 2007. Meanwhile, I am accepting the things I cannot change. Progress is incremental. Chemotherapy has left my muscles and ligaments stiff and sore. I have lymphedema, which is exacerbated by heat, salt, and repetitive motions, including spending too much time at my computer keyboard. Every day I look for the courage to change the things I can. I can't run, but I can swim—not well or for very long, but even a few minutes of swimming or exercising in the water really help with the swelling in my arm. I had thought that swimming during radiation was a no-no, but my research has indicated that it's fine to swim as long as I stay moisturized and stop if radiation burns cause the skin to break.

I was tempted to try an aquafit class at my local YMCA, but was put off by the idea of being bald and one-breasted in an exercise class. I enlisted my mother-in-law and went anyway. It seemed that everyone was too busy exercising to pay attention to me, and I was too busy concentrating on the exercises to feel self-conscious. It was a good workout. Tonight my arms are that good kind of sore.

At the end of the class, a woman came up to me in the showers and said, "We're part of the same club." She finished treatment eleven years ago.

It turns out that someone did notice me. I'm glad.

It Ain't Contagious

Cancer makes some people very uncomfortable. Even some folks I know fairly well clearly find it hard to meet my eye or spend any time in my presence since I started undergoing treatment.

They should be a bit more like my friend Shawn. I had beer and nachos with him and a couple of other friends last Friday night. Although we've been in regular contact, it was the first time we'd seen each other since I went on leave from work in January. At one point I commented that I was feeling pretty full and sleepy. "Don't pass out!" he admonished. "We'll take a marker and write stuff on your head!"

I really believe it's better to put it all out there, and if you can make me laugh in the process, so much the better.

Tomorrow, I go under the beam. I'll write soon about what is bound to be a surreal experience.

Overwhelmed

Too much to think about—new experience, new information to absorb. I had been warned that the mind can go to a pretty scary place when the door closes on the radiation room and the buzzing starts.

It's too soon to feel the effects of the beam, and each session lasts for only a few minutes. I find it hard, though, not to lie there and ponder what these rays could be doing to my body, and to consider my own mortality. It is, after all, a bit of a mind-fuck that the treatment for cancer is in itself carcinogenic.

I'm fine, though, really. And the radiation therapists are really nice.

Twenty-three radiation sessions to go.

I think it's time to curl up with a bowl of ice cream and a good murder mystery while I listen to my dog snore on the couch beside me.

39

Sounds like a fake age, doesn't it? But today is really, truly my thirty-ninth birthday.

Thirty-nine things I have learned this year (in no particular order):

1. Sometimes all it takes is a bit of initiative to create change in an unpleasant situation.

2. Most people will surprise you with their goodness and generosity, which is especially helpful to remember in today's disturbing global context.

3. I have a greater capacity to forgive than I thought I did.

4. It is possible to fall in love all over again.

5. Children, no matter how sensitive, are surprisingly resilient.

6. My children are lovely human beings. Okay, so I knew that already, but the boys have been tested this year and have impressed me in countless ways.

7. Laughter really is the best medicine.

8. I am loved. I knew that before, but now I can feel it in my bones.

9. I really do have a nicely shaped head.

10. I continue to be an optimist at heart.

11. I am also, as a friend said when I was first diagnosed, "a tough customer."

12. I should feel proud of my strength and positive outlook; they are getting me through treatment in better shape than many cancer patients.

13. I can do anything I set my mind to do.

14. I don't have to do everything just because I can.

15. Somewhat paradoxically, admitting vulnerability makes me stronger.

16. As youth is wasted on the young, good health is wasted on the fit. I didn't know enough to appreciate good health until my health was seriously threatened.

17. Sadness and joy can be inextricably mixed.

18. Someone I love told me a few months ago that I had impossibly high expectations of those who care for me. Just because someone cannot do one thing I ask or expect does not mean that he or she does not love me or that he or she is rejecting me. She was right. This was a very important lesson for me to learn.

19. Trusting is not a sign of weakness, nor is distrust a way to protect myself from getting hurt (see above).

20. It is okay to ask for help when I need it.

21. Red and blue are my two favourite colours. Passion and peace, activity and reflection. These are things I require in equal measures.

22. A pedicure is good therapy.

23. Exercise is a panacea.

24. There is no perfect way to support someone in crisis. Whatever feels right to you will probably be the right thing.

25. I am less judgmental than I used to be.

26. I will never be a religious person.

27. Very sick or severely disabled people used to scare me. They still do, but I know how to get past my fears.

28. My own fears help me understand why some people are now uncomfortable being around me.

29. It is fortunate that I was in the best physical shape of my life when I was diagnosed with cancer. I was the only woman in my arm of the clinical trial who was not admitted to hospital during treatment. My doctors think this is because I was mentally tough and physically fit.

30. I love to write and I'm good at it.

31. Being patient is very hard work, but worth the rewards.

32. Life is too short for pettiness.

33. Having a life-threatening illness is not as scary as I feared it would be.

34. A missed opportunity is not a disaster. Life is full of opportunity if one is open to it.

35. It is infinitely easier to be sick and middle class than sick and poor.

36. Medicare works.

37. There is a cancer club. None of us would have chosen to join, but we understand each other in a way that no one else can.

38. I have a very good life.

39. I still have a great deal left to learn.

Cancer and Me

A few days ago, I attended a Melissa Etheridge concert. It was an amazing show. The woman is a wonderful musician and songwriter who performed with great energy for more than two hours.

And she's a cancer survivor. In fact, she discovered her lump when she was last in Ottawa in 2004. Her return to this city must have felt triumphant. I have always been a fan of her music, but the way she handled cancer and what she wrote about the experience have turned her into one of my heroes. Her description of chemotherapy really resonated with me. It's hard not to feel a kinship with someone whose experiences so closely reflect my own.

I have listened to her music a lot during treatment—her old songs, to which I know all the words, and some new ones, recorded more recently, that can bring tears to my eyes or make the hair on the back of my neck stand up.

It was quite wonderful to see her on stage, obviously strong, fit, and joyous.

There was, however, a moment during the concert that has given me much to think about. Melissa talked about the brutality of chemo and the love and support of her spouse and community that got her through it. She also talked about how cancer made her re-examine her life and rethink her priorities. These things are true for me as well. Then she summed up her experience by saying, "Cancer is a gift." That's when she lost me.

There is no question that there are ways in which having cancer has enhanced my life. I am stronger and more confident. I am also much more cognizant of what a fortunate person I am. I have benefited greatly from the time I've had to reflect over the last few months.

But would I say that cancer is a gift? Am I glad that it happened to me? Absolutely not. I am still furious.

Not long after my diagnosis, I purchased a T-shirt that more accurately reflects my feelings. It has the letters CCKMA emblazoned on the front, with the smaller caption: "Cancer can kiss my ass."

In Perspective

I was going through some papers today, looking for information on lymphedema, when I found some notes summarizing the results of the tests performed on my tumours.

I've been so bogged down in the grind of treatment and its side effects that I sometimes lose perspective on why I am doing this. This was a worthwhile, if chilling, reminder to revisit the medical big picture.

The pathologists, from whom I had asked for an informal second opinion, explained that I had a "high-grade tumour and very aggressive cancer." They also advised me that I probably had dormant cells elsewhere in my body, since my cancer cells "showed an inherent characteristic of dissemination," as was evident from the fact that I had positive lymph nodes and, by the time of surgery, palpable tumours under my arms. Their final words of advice were, "Don't hold back thinking you'll have multiple ways to come back at this. Assume this is your best shot now."

And that is why I am putting myself through all this. Aggressive cancer means aggressive treatment. As my friend Andrea said, in a very loving message she sent me in February, "Cancer is bad, but we will be badder." And we have been.

Good to Be Here

I ran into a group of friends yesterday, one of whom I hadn't seen in a long time. When she said that it was nice to see me, I replied, "It's good to be here."

My friend Cathy, who was in my shoes two years ago, said, "It means a whole lot more than it used to, doesn't it?" It does indeed. It's good to be here.

■ **Wednesday, August 23, 2006**

A Conversation

As I sat waiting for my family to pick me up outside the cancer centre yesterday, I was approached by an elderly woman who had been sitting on the next bench.

"You have beautiful skin," she said. I was, of course, thrilled at the compliment as I have been feeling anything but beautiful lately.

She asked if I was in treatment at the centre. I said that I was.

"I have lung cancer," she said. "I never smoked, but I worked in intelligence. I worked mostly with men. The rooms we met in would be blue with smoke."

"And also, the spy planes brought in films taken overseas, which I handled regularly," she continued. "They had a coating on them. My colonel says he wouldn't be surprised if that's what caused the cancer as several others we worked with also have it."

I told her that I have breast cancer. She replied that her sister had breast cancer and is doing well, but is nervous as she approaches the five-year mark.

"I have lung cancer," she repeated. "And it's not the good kind of lung cancer. I'm thinking of going to San Antonio, Texas. There is a doctor there.... They can cure cancer now, but if the drugs don't make money, then the drug companies won't sell them. And the doctors here, they won't do anything that isn't in the medical mainstream. I think I'll go, but I need to find out more. I shouldn't say this, but I have lots of money. Still, I want to make sure they aren't quacks. I looked the place up on the Internet and it looks good. I have a brother who is a doctor in Victoria. I'm going to get him to look into it, but I think I'll go.... So many people have cancer now."

She paused to look at the book in my lap. "What are you reading?" (It was *The Lighthouse* by P.D. James.)

"I haven't read that one. She's not my favourite. Well, her stories are okay, but as a person.... " (Makes a face)

"Are you waiting for a ride?" I ask her.

(Laughs) "Yes, my daughter. She drives an old jalopy. It's a wreck. She has a million-dollar house, but still drives that thing. She's not a show-off, that's for sure."

"Such beautiful skin," she says again, and reaches out to stroke my face.

I go back to my book, and shortly after, her daughter pulls up in a battered blue Toyota Camry, with the windows rolled down. She waves goodbye as she gets in the car.

I liked her. I wonder how much of her story was true.

■ Monday, August 28, 2006

Grumpy

I am burned and tired and just plain fed up. Only six more radiation
treatments to go.

Sometimes It's Hard

I'm a bit of a mess these days. I've got a very bad radiation burn that is blistered and oozing, and I've been afflicted with a fatigue that defies description. A bit dramatic that, no?

So it's not surprising, I guess, that my emotions are all a little close to the surface. I was especially feeling it earlier in the week. Frustration, the effects of treatment, the time I've lost to cancer, and the ramifications of battling a life-threatening illness ... it all hit me with the force of a tidal wave.

I'm feeling quite a bit better now, though. I spent the week doing as little as I could. Resting, reading. I even had a friend come with me to radiation. This had been planned for a while, but the timing could not have been better.

Tim and the boys have gone away for the weekend. Last night they saw *Spamelot* in Toronto. Today, Sacha and Tim are taking part in the year's most highly anticipated event—a comic book convention. Before leaving, Sacha hugged me and said, "Don't die while we're gone."

I started to reprimand him and then realized that he wasn't joking. He asked me, "There isn't a chance, is there, that you could die before I come back?"

I reassured him that the cancer treatment was to make sure that all the cancer was out of my body. "And you know what? If it ever does come back, we'll treat it again."

"So does this mean that we don't have to worry for at least a year?"

"Yes," I answered.

He looked so relieved.

Sometimes, I hate how hard this is.

Bizarre

Cancer treatment is a very strange thing. The purported cures come with a whole host of side effects that I'm convinced are not fully understood by anyone.

I know a woman who was travelling abroad to celebrate the end of treatment. One day, she noticed that her treated breast had turned brown. On her return home, she consulted her radiation oncologist, who insisted that this change could not have been brought on by treatment. She raised the subject with an alternative practitioner, who said, "Don't ask your doctors. Ask other women." The next time her support group met, this woman mentioned what had happened to her breast. Four of the twelve women in the group had experienced the same thing. None had told their doctors. Brown breasts, blistered skin, blackened toenails, and bald heads.

Sometimes I think we haven't come that far since medieval doctors sought to cure the plague with bloodletting and poultices made from human excrement.

The Last Time

Today, I will go for radiation for the last time.

I'll enter the cancer centre and turn right at the door marked "Radiotherapy," scan my card to get in the queue, go and change into my robes (one backwards and one open at the front), and sit in the waiting room.

When my name is called, I will go and lie on a table that has been set up just for me. I'll slip out of one of my robes, let the other fall open, lift my knees so they can put a cushion under them, and tuck my left hand under hip. My right arm will go over my head and into a special brace. I won't move again until the end of treatment.

The therapists will spend some time making sure I am aligned perfectly, with the help of lasers, lines they have drawn on me with permanent marker, and the five little tattoos I was given before I started treatment. When they are satisfied that everything is set up the way it should be, they will drape something called a bolus (pliable plastic-like material that draws the rays to the skin's surface; treatment will be interrupted partway through to remove it) across my chest. Then they will turn off the lights and leave the room. The door will close with an audible click, a green light will turn to red, and treatment will begin.

The machine they use looks like a giant lamp, with jaws at its centre that open and close to control the amount of radiation emitted. As it moves around me, it makes a whirring noise and a high-pitched buzzing with each dose.

It will take only a few minutes to treat my back, chest, axilla (underarm), and clavicle. This felt like so much longer during the first week of treatment when I was still freaked out about being treated with radiation.

Then the therapists will come in, I'll say "thank you," and be on my way. I might cry.

Radiation was a pretty dehumanizing process. As a coping mechanism, I deliberately engaged the radiation therapists, asking questions or making observations. I am very grateful to the therapists and nurses who took the time to respond and who treated me as a whole person and not just body parts to be treated. I hope they realize what an enormous difference this made.

More Than Skin Deep

The stages of recovery from radiation:

1. Burned, blistered, raw, achy, and sore.

2. Fragile and sensitive.

3. Renewal. Still very tender, but on the road to healing.

4. Better. Not as new, but strong, healthy, and fit.

I am hovering somewhere between stages 3 and 4, sometimes taking two steps forward and one step back. I am making progress, though. My skin is healing, too.

Part Two

Reclaiming My Old Life

Seeking Balance

Apparently, people on long-term disability don't often call their insurance company to ask, "Can I go back to work now?" At least that's what my insurance rep told me when I spoke with her.

"What's the rush?" asked my oncologist when I mentioned a return to work.

And there certainly are many other things with which I could fill my time and not get bored, aside from physiotherapy and trying to find my house under all the rubble.

I know how lucky I am to have a supportive employer with a good insurance plan. I am also very grateful that I live in Canada, where we have socialized medicine (women without health insurance face alarmingly high death rates), and have a terrific oncologist who supports whatever choice I need to make as long as I promise to take things slowly.

In part, I want to return to work slowly so I can build up my stamina gradually and not feel overwhelmed by the shock of trying to get up to speed.

But that's not all. I attended a staff retreat last week at the Chateau Montebello, in a village near where I grew up. I'd always dreamed of staying there. The truth is, I felt energized by the experience and, in fact, have continued to have more energy since my return. It was so good to be around people and to have my thoughts be consumed by something other than cancer for a while.

I love my work, and my co-workers were an enormous source of support during treatment. And a significant part of my identity has always come from my work life.

I am a mother, lover, friend, trade unionist, and now, irrevocably (but not primarily), a cancer patient. Each of these identities is important to me and I need to give voice to each of them in order to feel whole.

I know that I need to be careful. The last thing I want is to end up on sick leave again, and labour movement jobs are famous for being demanding and stressful. I am going to have to set clear boundaries and figure out how to pace myself.

But I feel ready to start reclaiming the life I had before cancer.

Not Enough to Think Pink

Pink is not my new favourite colour unless it's hot pink; then maybe we can talk.

I will never, ever, buy a pastel pink sweater with pink ribbons on the buttons just because "a portion of the proceeds" goes to breast cancer research.

I resent large corporations benefiting from breast cancer and find the small donations made by some to be tantamount to fraud, but I knew there was more to my extreme annoyance than this (and the fact that very many breast cancer baubles are hideously ugly).

And then I had a conversation that had nothing to do with breast cancer.

I was in my local fair-trade coffee shop the other day buying beans. I ordered Brazilian, their very darkest roast, and was informed that it would not be available for several months. "Do you want to know why?" asked the clerk.

She told me that a big-box chain store had decided they wanted to start a fair-trade line of coffee and had bought out all the beans from the co-op in Brazil. Shortly afterwards, they cancelled these plans, leaving the co-op farmers to reach out again to their smaller distributors.

That a large multinational wants in is a testament to the power of the fair-trade consumer, but that this low-wage, anti-union, sweat-shop-supporting behemoth should hop on the fair-trade bandwagon is beyond hypocritical.

And that, I realized, is what bugs me about breast cancer product promotions. Too often the products sold are full of carcinogens or are made under conditions that are highly toxic to the environment. I don't want any part of that.

Let's make our donations directly to organizations that are working to prevent, treat, and cure breast cancer.

Gifts That Cancer Gave Me

I continue to maintain that cancer is not a gift. It is an evil scourge and I am still really pissed off that I got it.

But someone asked me this evening if I write every day and I said, "Yes. That's the gift that cancer gave me."

Here, in fairness to cancer, are some other things it gave me, which doesn't mean I'm not still working on kicking its ass:

1. The knowledge that humour can be found in the darkest places.

2. A renewed appreciation for the people who love me.

3. A sense of confidence in myself and my ability to face new and tough challenges.

4. Perspective.

5. An abiding love for dark, dark chocolate dipped in green tea.

Not Much Left

It's a rainy day in Ottawa and I am fighting off the cold my young son brought into the house. I feel like fixing myself a nice comforting, healthy snack. But the question of what to eat is not one that is easily answered.

I've been reading (or rather skimming the chapter summaries of) *Foods That Fight Cancer: Preventing Cancer through Diet*. It is, all in all, a positive book, full of beautiful pictures of leafy greens, bright citrus, and even lovely dark chocolate and red wine. However, the author's list of foods to avoid leaves me cold:

- Fried foods (fair enough)

- Processed foods (makes sense)

- Red meat (in excess)

- Alcohol (in excess)

- Smoked foods (ack!!!)

- Marinated foods (double-ack!!!)

I understand that this is not so terribly restrictive, but add to this the "foods to avoid" list from the very helpful information session that I attended this week on lymphedema management and prevention:

- Processed and refined foods

- Coffee (oh no!!)

- Alcohol (bye, bye red wine)

- Sugar

- Saturated fats

- Red meat

- Dairy

- Chocolate (so much for my daily guilt-free fix)

- Salty foods (no more Vietnamese noodle soup?)

- Spicy foods (might as well eat Pablum for the rest of my life)

"What's left?" I ask you. Fruit, vegetables, water, flaxseed.

Okay. Going to make vegetable soup now. I'm going to use broth with salt, though, because it's all I've got and, as the lymphedema trainer said, "You've still got to live your life."

Where I'm at

In mid-September I had a heart scan. This is the test where they inject you with radioactive material, wait twenty minutes, then take video of your heart, pumping away. I got to watch a little bit of it and, as far as I could tell, my heart seemed to be doing a very good job.

A week or so later, I went to see my medical oncologist, expecting to be given a date to start Herceptin. Instead, I was told that my heart had not sufficiently recovered from chemo.

The chemo I had was pretty aggressive, and there is always a 1–2 percent chance that chemo will permanently damage your heart. There is also a 1–2 percent chance that Herceptin will damage the heart. If the two drugs are taken too close together, there is a 30 percent chance of the heart being permanently damaged. Chemo is very, very toxic, and Herceptin, which I will be taking every three weeks for a year, is pretty toxic, too.

My next heart scan is scheduled for November 10 and I hope to start Herceptin shortly thereafter. My heart and head should both be ready by then.

I have an appointment with my radiation oncologist this morning. My skin seems to have recovered really well and I am working hard at regaining strength and mobility in my shoulder and arm. I expect to be told that I am doing well, but I admit that I'm nervous. I am making good progress, though, and as my hair grows, I look more like a hedgehog than a cancer patient.

I think I have reached the point where it is not immediately obvious that I've been in chemotherapy. A highlight of the staff retreat

I attended a couple of weeks ago was the moment a colleague from Vancouver, who doesn't know me well, inquired as to what kind of leave I'd been on. That made me feel really good.

Not Bloody Likely

My radiation oncologist always treats me as if I am about to burst into hysterical tears. It makes me crazy.

When I start to show annoyance, he seems to take this as further evidence of potential instability and it only makes him worse. I am trying to learn to keep my mouth shut, get the information I need, and get out of there, but it's not easy.

On the other hand, yesterday's appointment held no nasty surprises. My skin is healing well and so is the rest of me, slowly but surely. Still working on patience, though.

Why Breast Cancer Isn't Sexy

I loathe my prosthesis. I have entertained fantasies about attacking it with a knife and watching its silicone innards ooze all over the floor.

I hate how it feels. I hate the way that it never looks quite right. I hate that I have to wear it. (Actually, mostly I don't wear it.) And I know I need to work at a solution as I don't want the first thing that people notice to be my missing breast and all it represents.

There has been much good feminist writing about the hype surrounding Breast Cancer Awareness month. I join these women in their condemnation of the commercialization of breast cancer, and I certainly don't believe that one form of cancer is more worthy of support than another.

But a couple of writers have referred to breast cancer as "sexy."

It wasn't so long ago that breast cancer was considered shameful—a secret to be protected. For many women, this is still the case. After all, breasts are still not something we talk about at the dinner table, in the boardroom, or in most day-to-day situations.

My breasts have variously been a source of embarrassment, shame, confusion, pleasure, and pride. Now I have only one, and a big scar where the other one used to be. I thought long and hard about going public about my mastectomy, and I decided that if I am to write honestly about my experience, this enormous source of discomfort, frustration, and sadness must be included.

Breast cancer mutilates a highly sexualized, commercialized, and central part of women's bodies. It is also a major cause of lymphedema, a further strain on our bodies, emotions, and sexual selves.

I hate my prosthesis. I hate what it represents.

Self-confidence is sexy. So is love. Power can be a turn-on. So are broad shoulders, a quick wit, and a sense of humour. Sometimes I am sexy.

Breast cancer will never be "sexy."

■ **Wednesday, November 1, 2006**

The Here and Now

It's not that cancer has turned me into a happier person. It is true, however, that I now experience joy differently. I have a renewed sense of the pleasure in the little things and, to my great surprise, a much greater ability to live in the moment.

I just spent a near-perfect weekend attending the theatre and tasting wine. I stayed at a lovely bed-and-breakfast with my sweetie. We had so much fun.

Life is full of so many interesting people and fun things to do.

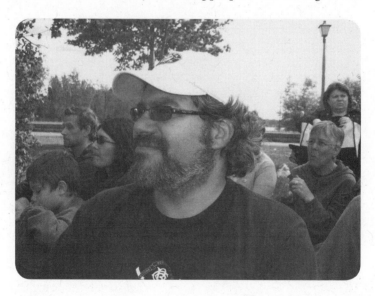

Back to Work

As reported a couple of weeks ago, I have begun to ease back into work. This is how it's been going:

October 16, meeting 1:30–4:30 p.m.

Spend morning on computer.

Take dog out for abbreviated walk.

Realize I am running late. Run through shower.

Take taxi to meeting, arrive late, sweaty, dishevelled, prosthesis askew.

Realize I have forgotten to eat. Spend meeting fighting to concentrate.

My friend Helen comments on how energized I seem. I am not energized. I am hysterical.

Spend next day in bed.

October 24, meeting 2:00–4:00 p.m.

Spend morning on computer.

Take dog out for abbreviated walk.

Call boss to say that I will be late. Find out that meeting is half an hour later than I thought it was.

Run through shower.

Take taxi to meeting, arrive just in time, looking slightly more pulled together than on previous occasion.

Actually pay attention in meeting.

Spend next day in bed.

October 31, office 9:30 a.m.–12:30 p.m.

Get kids off to school and daycare. Run around trying to find various
   things I need to take to work.

Spouse drives me to work; arrive five minutes late.

Dump stuff in office, spend morning feeling completely overwhelmed, not sure what to do first.

Go home. Sleep for two hours.

November 2, office 9:30 a.m.–12:30 p.m.

Drop off son on the way into work.

Arrive 15 minutes early.

Attend meeting, manage to pay attention *and* participate.

Meet with the occupational therapist sent by the insurance company
   to assess my work space.

Spend last half hour sorting through files, go home, do homework
   for writing class, and walk dog.

I'd call that progress, wouldn't you?

Ouch

I had way too much fun last night. A group of friends and co-workers took part in World Trivia Night, an annual event that is always a blast.

Chemo brain was not too much in evidence, although I am not convinced there were any questions to which I was the only one from my team to have the answer. However, it's not the trivia that is causing my hangover.

I like wine—a lot. However, it is highly unusual for me to have more than a glass or two with dinner (and that, only a couple of times a week). Last night, I had this tiny little plastic wine glass and it just kept getting refilled (note my use of the passive tense here). I was thirsty. The wine tasted good. I had a really good time.

Today, however, I have my very first hangover in a very long time.

Funny thing, the same spouse who was unbelievably sweet, caring, and sympathetic during chemo was most decidedly unsympathetic when I was dragging my ass around this morning. (Okay, so it was noon and he was making french toast and cleaning up the kitchen at the same time.)

Go figure.

At Least I Roasted a Chicken

The path to recovery from cancer treatment is certainly neither straight nor flat. In fact, if I were training on a path like this one, I'd have some serious thighs of steel.

My commitment to taking good care of myself has been somewhat inconsistent. Some days I eat really well. Today, I roasted a chicken, an experience that gave new meaning to the phrase "It takes a village"—or, in this case, a good friend on the phone and an Internet search. Some days, nary a vegetable crosses my lips.

Some days I manage a long, vigorous walk and my strength-training exercises (key to strengthening my arm and relieving the pain in my shoulder). Some days, the end of the day rolls around and I have barely left the couch.

My return to work has felt a little bumpy as well. Today, I worked on an assignment I was asked to do last week. I had it almost finished when I left. I am working three hours, two mornings a week for the first month. Later this afternoon, I found out that a colleague had started work on the same little project. And I realized that what I had done was *wrong*.

This totally bummed me out.

But I roasted that chicken today. "Do I need to do anything to the vegetables before I throw them in?" "Which end of the chicken is the neck?" "What do the innards look like?" "Will the house burn down if I take a walk while it's cooking?" Thank goodness for my friend Helen, even if she couldn't stop laughing. That's something.

And I haven't missed a walk in more than a week.

When I finish this post, I'll clean up the kitchen, and then I will do my exercises.

I don't really have the choice of giving up or, to beat a metaphor to death, of leaving the path I'm on, though some days I need to just plop myself down in the dirt and have a good vent about how hard this can be. I have to keep putting one foot in front of the other and hopefully, as time goes on, those hills will feel a little less steep.

Pain and My Inner Selves

I'm in a bit of pain today. My shoulder is very tight, having been damaged by surgery and radiation. It's become much worse in the last couple of weeks. My massage therapist and physiotherapist have both reassured me that if I keep doing my exercises, the ache will go away, and reaching for a glass from the cupboard will no longer take my breath away.

I also have a stitch in my upper right abdomen. It feels much worse if I stand up, cough, or breathe deeply. My spouse thinks it's a pulled muscle (from the above-mentioned exercises). My inner hypochondriac, aided and abetted by the Internet, would have me be worried about pancreatitis, gallstones, or worse. I have decided to ignore my inner hypochondriac.

I know that lots of people deal very stoically with living in constant pain. I've been feeling some newfound empathy and respect for these people. My pain is very likely to go away in short order. Not knowing if this would ever be the case would be very hard indeed. Today, though, I am nursing my inner wuss, taking it easy, and waiting for the pain to subside.

Some Things Are Easy

The phone rang this morning. The caller ID showed the school's number. I grabbed it, and went on to have the following conversation:

SACHA, AGE EIGHT: (Tearful) "You forgot the refreshments for the party!" (They were having a class party as a reward for good behaviour.)

ME: "I can bring you cheesies." (Lest you judge me, the last time there was a party, we sent homemade granola bars. All but one—eaten by the teacher—came home again.)

SACHA: "Okay. You can bring my agenda, too."

ME: "Okay."

SACHA: "And my POW." ("Problem of the week," a weekly homework assignment that had been completed on Monday.) "It's the only thing I haven't handed in."

ME: "Is there anything else you might need?"

SACHA: "Let's see. You could bring in a CD of dance music."

ME: (Silence)

SACHA: "Wait a second. Are you being sarcastic?"

ME: "I am being sarcastic, but I'll bring you a CD."

And I did.

Paging Dr. Jung

I had a dream last night that the cancer came back, or rather that it had never really left.

I'd had a test of some sort and it revealed that I had tumours in my chest and abdomen. There was nothing I could do to make it go away; just eat well and take good care of myself. And it was sort of implied that the cancer had metastasized (spread, invaded, colonized) because I hadn't been taking good care of myself.

Not that hard to deconstruct. Where my consciousness fears to tread, my subconscious takes me.

I Don't Get It

A couple of weeks ago, my son came home with what looked like orange marker on his arm. We were curious.

ME: "Why do you have orange marker on your arm?"

SACHA: "I was trying to make a wound."

ME: "A wound."

TIM: (Simultaneously) "Cool! After your homework is done, we can work on making it look more authentic."

It's amazing what you can do with red food colouring, petroleum jelly, and cloves.

Thank you, Y chromosome.

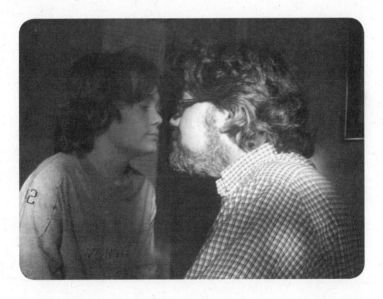

His Version of Reason

MY THREE-YEAR-OLD SON, DANIEL, CLUTCHING HIS ARM: "My ankle hurts!"

ME: "That's your elbow."

DANIEL: "No! My ankle hurts!"

ME: "That's your elbow, honey."

DANIEL: "No! My ankle hurts!"

ME: (pointing to his ankle) "This is your ankle."

DANIEL, CLUTCHING HIS ANKLE: "My ankle hurts!"

Building My Vocabulary

I love words, and I love learning new ones.

Just after I went on leave to start treatment, a friend got me hooked on online Scrabble.

There are, however, words that I have learned in the last year that have not given me pleasure:

Adenocarcinoma. Lymphedema. Metastatic. Especially metastatic, a word I didn't know a year ago that I now think about every day.

What's the old rule for learning a word? Use it five times and it's mine for life?

Hospital Fashion

I've written before about the indignity of hospital robes. In my experience, they are hideous, never fit right, and just generally add to the vulnerability you experience as a patient.

Then I discovered the three-armhole robe.

It's a really neat design, and they actually had detailed instructions as to how to put it on taped to the changing-room wall. Left arm. Right arm. Then bring it around to the front and put the left arm through the third hole. Comfortable, modest, and stays put without ties. It was a truly ugly yellow-green colour, though. I guess when it comes to hospital gowns (and many other things in life), you can't have it all.

The Raven and the Sun

This summer, I was out enjoying the sunshine toward the end of a chemo cycle and I stopped in at a jewellery store to browse. I spotted some lovely rings, designed and crafted by Native artists from the West Coast.

My favourites were silver with the animals of Haida legend in gold. None of the rings fit me, but the staffperson who showed me the rings said that the artists would do custom work if I wanted to give some thought as to which animal I wanted.

It didn't take long for me to realize that I loved the story of the raven, who put the sun, the moon, and the stars back in the sky after the world had gone dark. The imagery, as I viewed the light at the end of my own tunnel, really captured my feelings of hope and joy at the thought of having put cancer treatment behind me.

I put in my order. I had no particular requests of the artist I had chosen (Joe Descoteaux), mentioning only to the clerk at the store that I loved the story of the raven and the sun.

The ring arrived on my birthday, several weeks earlier than I had been told to expect, and it is beautiful. It is also very special. The artist designed my ring with a raven with the sun in his beak, about to return it to the sky. I love it.

Just as the raven is very tricky, so also is fate. My life is taking some twists and turns that I did not plan for when I ended treatment. My ring, however, still symbolizes hope and joy to me, as well as all the good things that bring light into my life every day.

Part Three

Metastasis, or "Worst Case Scenario"

■ **Monday, November 27, 2006**

Metastatic

November 9: I wake up with a stitch on my right side. I figure that I had either pulled a muscle doing abdominal exercises or that I'm coming down with something. I take the day off work.

The week of November 12: The pain has intensified a little and I am plagued by the "gut-rats," an expression I coined during my pregnancies to describe the intestinal discomfort I felt. I take a pregnancy test—negative, thank gawd. My doctor had warned that chemopause would not necessarily make me infertile and that even if it did, that state of affairs was unlikely to be permanent. Toward the end of that week, I call to make an appointment with my family doctor.

November 18: It occurs to me that I might be showing symptoms of Celiacs Disease, an auto-immune disease that causes an inability to digest gluten. My sister has it, and it tends to run in families. I groan and cross my fingers. Celiacs would be a pain.

November 19: Returning from a walk with my son, I have an attack of the most intense abdominal pains I have experienced since giving birth. It occurs to me that I might have something more serious than Celiacs with which to contend. I notice for the first time that my waist seems to have disappeared and the area on my right side between my waistband and rib cage is hard and swollen.

November 21: My GP examines me. When she asks me to take a deep breath, I yelp in pain. Obviously distressed, she tells me that my liver is very enlarged. She says, "I'm sorry. I know that's not what you wanted to hear." That's an understatement. In the last few days, I have learned that when breast cancer metastasizes (spreads to areas of the body other than the breast or nearby lymph nodes), it most often goes to the bones, chest, brain, lungs, or liver. My GP calls the nurse who works with my medical oncologist, and urges them to schedule an ultrasound as soon as possible. I go from the appointment to my hair salon, where I get my hair cut and dyed red in defiance.

November 22: I have a previously scheduled appointment with my medical oncologist, although I end up seeing the GP who works with him. It is clear that she, too, is very worried. She orders blood work and says that they will get me in for an ultrasound before the end of the week. She does say that other conditions can cause a painful swelling of the liver, and that they will test for those things as well. As we are leaving, Tim and I agree that when you are hoping to test positive for hepatitis, life has become very weird.

November 23: The blood test results are in. My liver functions are elevated. Everything else is fine. I am scheduled for an ultrasound later that day.

November 24: I have a late-afternoon appointment with the oncologist. We wait a long time. My knees buckle when the nurse comes for me. I know that I am about to hear bad news. My oncologist enters, grim-faced. He is compassionate, but doesn't sugar-coat things. I like him. He tells me that I have more tumours on my liver "than they could count." He tells me that from now on, we will not be talking about curing me, but extending my life and making me as comfortable as possible. The first thing I remember saying is, "I have two beautiful children!" and "I'm only thirty-nine years old," as though these things should exempt me.

My oncologist was wonderful, clear, and, as I said before, very compassionate. I finally screwed up the courage to ask, "How long do I have? Weeks?"

"I'm better than that," he replied. I really loved that answer. Then he said, "Years. Not decades."

So I restart chemo, along with Herceptin, tomorrow. My heart has still not recovered as much as my oncologist would like from the chemo, but, as you can tell by the timeline above, my cancer is aggressive and fast-moving. We need to act now.

The good news is that the new chemo drug I'll be taking is less hard on the body and less likely to cause nausea and hair loss. I may also be able to avoid taking the steroids that I hated almost as much as the chemo.

I am, all things considered, in fairly good shape emotionally, and not just because I am full of morphine. I have lots going for me and I intend to revel in the good things, especially my wonderful community of family and friends.

Don't get me wrong. I am really, really pissed off, and I'm sure that the real emotional fallout is yet to come, but for now, I'm okay.

The Darkest Humour

November 24: Tim and I had just been told the news of my metastasis, which had been followed by a truly unhelpful session with the hospital social worker. As we were leaving the social worker's office, she handed us a parking pass, the first time either of us had seen such a thing.

We looked at the pass. We looked at each other.

ME: "What do you know! With every death sentence ..."

TIM: "You get to park for free."

A Wild Ride

Boy, Herceptin is a trip. One moment I was fine, the next I was flopping around like a fish, with my teeth clattering against my jaw. This lasted for several minutes. It was one of the most bizarre experiences of my life.

They used Demerol to stop the shaking. A lot of Demerol. I was very happy.

Then they told me I was running a fever.

After examining me and deciding there was no sign of an infection that could be causing the fever, the doctor decided that treatment could proceed.

We were at the hospital for eight long hours.

Apparently these are not uncommon side effects of Herceptin and I am less likely to experience them next time.

That's good news. I liked the Demerol, but I really didn't like the convulsing.

Celebrity

Apparently my reaction to Herceptin yesterday caused quite a bit of excitement at the cancer centre. The side effects I experienced—chills and shakes, followed by fever—are quite normal. It was the intensity of the reaction that set tongues wagging. My oncologist called it "dramatic." And the fact that I had to go back today was definitely unusual.

During the night, I got the shakes again, although they were much milder than on the previous morning. Then I got the fever, and it just kept climbing. It peaked at 40°C. By then, we were on our way back to the cancer centre.

They put me in bed, gave me IV fluids, drew some blood, gave me assorted pills for fever and pain, and I dozed on and off for a couple of hours. By the time the blood tests came back and I was released, I felt considerably better.

And the good news? My oncologist and the cancer centre pharmacist think I am reacting so intensely because the Herceptin is working really well. I like that.

The other good news? The side effects of Herceptin usually diminish significantly after the first round. Then again, I seem to be an unusual cancer patient.

Hi, Honey, I'm Home!

Dear blog:

Oh, how I've missed you.

Only four days in the hospital could keep my fingers from the keyboard. You should have seen how my hands trembled when my laptop and I were reunited. I hope it will provide some measure of comfort to you that I thought about you all the time while we were apart, composing entire missives during the nights' darkest hours.

The hospital stay was necessary due to fever and a dramatic drop in my white blood cells (I'll write more about that tomorrow), but it felt like such a long time to be away. And no, I did not ring for the nurse in the middle of the night to beg for the use of a computer with Internet access. But I thought about it.

While it would be untrue to say that I cease to exist without you (we did spend four days apart, after all), I do know that you help me to understand my thoughts and provide a venue for me to say the things I dare not speak aloud, even to myself. You are a reflection of me, a place for me to process my thoughts and figure out how life's events have made me feel. I promise to be faithful to you during the coming weeks, months, and years as we face the challenges life delivers to us.

Baby, I'm back, and I'm yours.
Love,
L.

Febrile Neutropenia

Sounds vaguely distasteful, doesn't it? Like something you wouldn't want your mother to know you'd contracted.

It's actually what happens when chemo beats the shit out of you and your white blood cells are pummelled out of existence, leaving you feverish and sleeping round the clock for days on end. At least that's what happened to me.

I was pretty stupid about it, actually. I had been told pretty clearly that if I had a fever that topped 38°C, I was to come into the hospital immediately. I didn't take my temperature for several days (and didn't think that I should be worried about sleeping all the time), and then when I did, I didn't think 38.4°C seemed all that high. (I was in grade school when Canada switched to metric and still prefer Fahrenheit for temperature. 38.4°C is 101°F.)

One cancelled chemo session and a four-day hospital stay on IV fluids and I can honestly say that I have learned my lesson. There's nothing like being in the hospital to help focus your thoughts. I was fortunate to have a private room, and even though my IV and I were permitted to wander the halls, I preferred to stay in the room. I was the only person on the oncology ward for febrile neutropenia; the other patients all appeared to be receiving palliative care. It terrified me.

I need to do everything I can to delay my own palliative stage of cancer treatment, and I need to come to terms with what it means to have a terminal illness. I'm working on it.

Through the Haze

I am ever so slightly stoned as I write this, having just taken a Tylenol 3. I call this the medium guns, as compared to morphine or the lovely high from Oxycontin. I have been trying to manage the pain with plain old extra-strength Tylenol, and usually that's fine, but sometimes I just need a little extra numbness.

I think my doctors actually think I'm pretty stoic. Speaking of doctors, I saw one of the GPs who works with my oncologist today. Dr. D. doesn't usually back up my oncologist, but I gather the place was really hopping. Dr. D. was also the doctor I saw during my recent hospital stay. I referred to her as the warden, and I definitely felt like I was in jail.

A couple of days into my stay, my friend Helen, who was visiting me when the doctor made her rounds, made a joke about how I was planning my escape. Dr. D. was most distinctly not amused. It took several minutes of reassurance from me before she stopped radiating disapproval.

Today's appointment went fairly well, though. My bone scan showed no evidence of metastasis. This means that although the cancer, having travelled from my breast, is likely elsewhere in my body, there appears to be no significant presence outside my liver. I've also been given the green light to start Herceptin and chemo again next Tuesday, pending blood test results. We need to make sure that those infection-fighting white blood cells have rebounded.

My heart has not yet recovered from the stress placed on it by my first six rounds of chemo (Taxotere, Adriamycin, and Cytoxan, known as TAC). However, the doctors have decided that given the aggressiveness of my cancer and the improvement I experienced after just one treatment, the benefits of Herceptin outweigh the risks (the big one being permanent heart damage). Consequently, though, I have regular echocardiograms, possibly heart medication, and a consultation with a cardiologist in my future.

Sigh.

Just a little over a year ago, I considered myself to be a very healthy person. Other than a brief stay in hospital when my second son was born (for his sake, not mine), I had only ever been hospitalized for a tonsillectomy when I was eight years old.

By the end of my appointment, though, I found that I had warmed to Dr. D. She may not smile much or laugh at my jokes, but it's clear that she is a caring doctor who wants to deliver good news. She did smile when I was finally sprung from hospital and when she delivered the news of my bone scan. She also is willing to take the time to answer questions and explain things without ever making me feel that she is "dumbing things down" or patronizing me. What's more, she is honest when she doesn't know the answer to a question, but quick to inform herself and get back to me.

I think this makes her a pretty good doctor.

This is life as a cancer patient: Full of surprises, not all of them bad.

Friday, December 15, 2006

I Melted

I went to the holiday concert at my son's school today.

His class was up first. Twenty-five eight-year-olds (all but four of them boys), all dressed in white shirts (except for one rebel in a grey sweatshirt), singing "Give Peace a Chance." As he first got on the stage, I could see that Sacha was scanning the crowd for me. I was sitting on the floor, having arrived a bit late. I got up on my knees and waved like a crazy woman. When he waved back, I blew him a kiss. Then, right there, on the stage, in front of his peers, he blew me a big kiss right back. It almost undid me. The performance was wonderful, and over very quickly.

An hour, several Christmas and Chanukah songs and a few poems later, we were done. After thanking his teacher, I went to collect him. We had planned to go to the movies, but instead, he asked to go home.

We cuddled up in the big chair in the basement, ate popcorn, and watched two episodes of "Buffy the Vampire Slayer."

I made him promise that he would never be too old to hug and kiss his Mama (except maybe in front of his friends).

Just Like My Mom

The concert I attended last Friday has got me thinking about the importance of these kinds of events in the lives of children and their parents. I was not feeling very well last Friday, but I knew how important it was to Sacha that I be there—how important it was to both of us.

I have very early memories of my mom driving a whole bunch of kids to dancing lessons. This started when I was very young (I remember us all being about five years old and my friend Philippe explaining to us how babies were made; I was afraid to kiss anyone for a long time after that) and continued through the early years of high school when I was mortified by our pea-green Torino with the rusted-out holes in the floor.

My mother would stay during the classes and cheer me on, encouraging me to work hard and do my best, but was also ready to take my side if she felt I was not being given the help or the credit she felt I deserved.

I also have a very clear memory of my mother coming on a field trip when I was in the early grades of elementary school. I was so proud to have her with us. And I recall how kind she was to a school friend of mine, a girl who had just lost her mother to cancer.

I don't think my mom ever felt acknowledged for the things she did for us on a daily basis—things like bringing my lunch to school when I forgot it, or letting me stay home to finish a project (it was a pioneer quilt; I had bitten off more than I could chew, but the end result was beautiful). It is only as an adult and a parent that I recognize the importance of these daily gestures as they told me that my accomplishments were important and so was I.

My parents' attendance took on a special importance when I was to take part in a performance of any kind. From Grade 8 Variety Night to annual dance recitals and innumerable school plays, I would always begin by scanning the crowd for their faces. It was so important to me that my parents be there to recognize my achievement.

Even before I was diagnosed with cancer, I would book off time to accompany my children on field trips as often as I could. And Tim and I make sure that one of us is always available to attend every classroom event, party, or presentation to which parents are invited.

The events of the last few months have made me feel even more strongly about showing up for my kids in this way. I do my very best to accept every invitation, attend every performance, no matter how brief or how peripheral my child's role.

I want to be there, and I want my kids to know their parents will do everything they can to watch them perform, present, read, or just show us their work.

I know how much this means to my kids because I know how much it meant to me.

Eventful Day

Blood tests.

Breakfast with friends.

Relatively painless Christmas shopping.

Chemo.

Throwing up.

Herceptin.

Teeth chattering, freezing, trembling mess, although it happened later in the treatment than last time and wasn't as intense.

Demerol and Gravol.

Sleep.

Kids woke me up when they returned from an outing with Grandma.

I'm running a fever again (38.5°C). Not going to emergency tonight (too full of sick people), but if the fever hasn't broken by morning, I am going back to the cancer centre.

I promise.

I'm Not in the Hospital

Although I have been there every day this week (today just for a CT scan and blood work).

The last few days have been a roller coaster, but I'm hanging in.

Oh, and yesterday I learned to give an orange an injection. Today I injected myself in the stomach. How cool is that?

I'm a Freakin' Pincushion

I had nine needles stuck into me for various reasons this week. I also learned how to inject myself in the belly with Neupogen, which I will now be doing for five days after each chemo treatment (that's ten days out of every three-week cycle).

It's weird jabbing yourself with a needle, but I can see how people get used to it. And I will do just about anything to bolster those infection-fighting, keeping-me-away-from-hospital-food white blood cells.

The last few days have been tough slogging, but I am home and my temperature has been normal for more than twelve hours so I am hopeful that all will be well through Christmas.

We lit the last Chanukah candle this evening. I think my oldest son may not sleep until Christmas. And my children were both especially lovely tonight.

It was nice to be reminded what joy feels like.

Another One down

We survived Christmas. There was lots of emotion, laughter, the usual family craziness, a few surprises, and an orgy of presents.

In our family, we open our presents to each other on Christmas Eve, a variation on the French-Canadian tradition. Santa comes during the night, so there are more presents (for the children) in the morning. We enjoy doing things this way, but it makes for a late night for the children *and* a very early morning.

We have now settled into the kids-are-home-what's-next? phase of the holidays. After all the visitors and presents, this period of relative quiet (no daycare and no school—sigh) feels a bit like a letdown to the kids and they are going a bit stir-crazy.

I had chemo yesterday, an event that was wonderfully uneventful. It was just the Vinorelbine (no Herceptin) and the whole process barely took ten minutes. Today, I'm a little green around the gills, but not nearly as sick as I was on the first go-round. This and the fact that I am in less pain today than I have been in weeks have put me in a very good mood.

The break from pain is incredibly welcome (an understatement) and I am choosing to take this change as a sign that the treatments are working and that my tumours are shrinking.

How I Do It

Someone asked me yesterday how I do it, meaning how I manage to keep it together in the face of my most recent diagnosis.

The truth is, sometimes I don't keep it together at all. There are moments when I feel like I'm standing on the edge of an abyss and it takes everything I have not to be pulled into the darkness. And at other times, I feel like I have fallen over the edge and just managed to pull myself out or, more often, have had someone who loves me grab my hand just in time.

And, even on the good days, there are hard moments, like the conversation I had today with my spouse about a call we need to make to our financial planner. We need to tell her that she will no longer need to put a plan together for my retirement. It's hard to say some things out loud.

But I do have so many good reasons to stay positive, to keep putting one foot in front of the other, willingly and with determination:

1. I want my kids to have an engaged, active mother. I plan to be around for some time yet and I want to enjoy my children. I also want them to remember me as strong, loving, and mostly happy.

2. There are still so many reasons to be happy. I went for my first post-treatment walk today. The sun was bright, the snow was new and white, and my dog's tail was wagging happily. What's not to enjoy?

3. I have so many people who love me (see above re. getting pulled out of the abyss), and have shown me in countless ways that they will never give up on me.

4. Life is full of fun surprises, like the gift certificate for amazon.ca that I found in my inbox the other day.

5. I still have lots to learn and do. Life is not boring, and with a lot of the petty stuff stripped away, many things are, in fact, more interesting.

6. The way I see it, I have two choices. I could wallow or I could choose to enjoy life as it is. I believe the latter route will help me to live longer and definitely make the time I have left more enjoyable. In a lot of ways, it just makes sense to choose to be positive.

I'm writing this from my brand spankin' new laptop. I needed a new one (and writing is so key to my happiness), but Santa went all out and got me a fancy one—100 GB hard drive! Whoo hoo! I've named her Betsy. She's beautiful.

Happy New Year, everyone

Looking up.

I had an appointment with the doctor who works with my oncologist today. I adore Dr. B. and today she was all smiles.

She says that it's her feeling, and that of Dr. G., my oncologist, that I am having these intense reactions to Herceptin because it's working. She says that they've seen these signs before when the treatment has been effective, and although the evidence is purely anecdotal, they are feeling very optimistic, and so am I. Cautiously optimistic, but optimistic all the same.

Consider the following:

1. The swelling in my liver has decreased somewhat dramatically. As recently as Christmas Day, I looked and felt like I had swallowed a watermelon. Both sides of my belly now look the same (which means like a woman who has had two kids and has never done a ton of ab work) and I can do up my pants. I can also go for walks (and I have been) without feeling like my insides are all mushed together.

2. I have not needed a painkiller stronger than extra-strength Tylenol since Boxing Day. Less than two weeks ago, I was on morphine.

3. My most recent blood test revealed that my liver functions have improved greatly since my diagnosis of metastasis.

It was nice to leave an oncology appointment with a smile on my face. I did have an echocardiogram again today (more on that tomorrow), the results of which may determine when I am next treated with Herceptin. The next session is scheduled for January 9, but the docs are concerned about the toll Herceptin might be taking on my heart, given the damage that has already been caused by Adriamycin, the "Red Devil" chemo drug that made me lose my hair.

I hope that I am given the green light to proceed (along with a couple of new drugs in the mix to reduce the intensity of my reactions). I am, of course, keen to keep attacking my tumours. I've been visualizing the chemo and Herceptin blasting the little bastards.

Dr. B. told me that she's ordering a new ultrasound to see what my liver looks like now that I've had a few treatments. She seems pretty confident that we'll see a marked improvement.

■ Thursday, January 4, 2007

A Hole in My Memory

I went for an echocardiogram yesterday at one of the local hospitals, one that does only testing and day surgery.

My mother-in-law took me to a CT scan at the same hospital on December 21. I remember discussing with her how quiet this hospital was and how much it had changed since my son was born there in 1998, when the hospital was less specialized. And I remember telling her that I had not been back there since that time.

When the technician asked, I told him I had been for an echo before at a different hospital (the one where most of my other tests have taken place and where the cancer centre is located), but I couldn't tell him when. He looked me up on the computer. I did go for an echo on December 4 at that very hospital, and he had been the technician who did it.

I remember none of it. The waiting room, reception, testing room, the test itself, or even the hospital—none of it seemed remotely familiar to me. I know that my friend Karin took me to the echo, but only because she returned my grey sweater a couple of weeks ago. I had noticed it was missing, but have no recollection of leaving it in her car.

I vaguely remember driving with Karin and mentioning that I was on morphine, which could be partially the cause of the hole in my memory, but nothing else. Mostly, I think my memory was impaired by the shock of hearing about and dealing with the diagnosis of metastasis and everything it means.

The human brain is really quite unfathomable.

So Far So Good

I had Herceptin yesterday, along with the Vinorelbine, the chemo I'm on. It's been more than twenty-four hours and I have not had a reaction to the Herceptin, nor am I running a fever.

The doctors had said that my reactions would probably diminish over time. To help matters along, they pumped me full of Demerol before treatment along with Gravol. (I've never taken a heavy-duty narcotic before when I wasn't in serious pain. What a trip!) I quickly became very stoned and very sleepy. They went on to give me the Herceptin very slowly (over ninety minutes) and then to keep me for an hour's observation.

It was a long day, but it was worth it. No chills, no shakes, no fever. I didn't write about this, but I landed in emergency the day after my last Herceptin treatment. Nothing like sitting in a waiting room full of coughing, puking people while your immune system is depressed. I'm pretty tired and a little green around the gills, but I've been able to read and sleep today.

It's a pretty gruelling routine I'm on in terms of the frequency of treatment, but the side effects (she says, crossing her fingers) seem to be less intense than those I experienced during the first go-round (before the metastasis). If I can eat a little, sleep, and read, everything is a little more bearable.

And I still have hair.

If I Knew Then ...

I should have taken out life insurance when I was healthy. My spouse and I were in the process of applying (had even gone through the physical exams) when I found my lump. I really, really wish we had acted sooner.

The Marvellously Mundane

At around 11:00 this morning, my little family piled into the station wagon and set off to run some errands. We went to the comic book store for my oldest son to spend a gift certificate—he and his father would have happily spent the whole day in the place—and then out for Vietnamese noodle soup. We were delighted to find our favourite *pho* soup in the middle of big-box store land.

Fortified, Daniel and I went grocery shopping at a store with little cars built into the carts, so Daniel could ride around in front and "drive," while my spouse and older son went to buy a new router for our network, ours having gone belly-up the day before. They met us before we were done and in time to help with the last bit of shopping.

Finally, we went to Canadian Tire. While Tim and little Daniel went in to buy skates, Sacha read comic books in the car and I returned a call to my parents. I was almost shocked into hanging up—my parents have acquired an answering machine. They are so thrilled with it that they are letting it pick up all incoming calls, even though it means they're on the hook for returning the long-distance call.

After the errands were done and we were home, I read Daniel a story while Tim put the groceries away. Next, I went for a walk with my friend Helen and my dog Jasper. We stopped for coffee and again for cat food. Tim and the boys went skating on a neighbourhood pond.

When I got home from the walk, a little chilled and, with the boys still out, I treated myself to a long, hot jasmine-scented bath and emerged feeling like I'd had a massage. Then I cleaned the kitchen while defrosting dinner (frozen chicken, frozen french fries, and frozen veggies, washed down with a freezing cold beer).

Does this all sound incredibly boring? I loved every minute of it. It seems that I have come to embrace the mundane, to revel in my ability to do normal things. And to feel that I've accomplished something.

I turned the chemo corner yesterday, feeling energetic and healthy. My next treatment is on Tuesday. I am savouring these few days when I feel like myself, eating, exercising, playing with my kids, and even buying groceries on a Sunday afternoon.

Wednesday, January 17, 2007

Pyjamas Again

Yesterday was a chemo day, so, of course, today was spent in my pyjamas. All things considered, I am doing well. I was really sick last night, but woke up at eleven this morning feeling tired, but only a little queasy. No Herceptin this time, only chemo.

My white blood cells, and in particular the infection-fighting neutrophils, have rebounded really well. My count yesterday was seven. I have no idea what this means, except that I was at zero when I was in the hospital, and at two a couple of weeks ago.

My echocardiogram showed that my heart is now functioning as well as it was before I was diagnosed with cancer. A little better, in fact. I can breathe easier now, knowing I won't be yanked off the Herceptin or forced to take heart medication.

I think this bodes well for my ultrasound on Friday. These things happen in threes, no?

By next week, I hope to tell you all the story of my incredible shrinking tumours.

Gut Feeling

I feel pretty lousy this evening. A few months ago, I would have chalked it up to a virus. I feel nauseated, bloated, and I have heartburn and other intestinal issues. This all started yesterday afternoon and has gradually worsened.

It's probably nothing, but I no longer have the confidence to feel that a cramp is just a cramp, nothing more. Hopefully I'll wake up tomorrow feeling much better.

I see the oncologist tomorrow afternoon. I'm also hoping that he has my ultrasound results and that our optimism has been well placed.

I'll let you know.

Moving in the Right Direction

My oncologist says that my gastrointestinal issues are nothing to worry about. Accordingly, I have told my inner hypochondriac to stand down.

He also said that my liver functions are now *normal*, repeating himself for emphasis and to make sure I grasped the import of this.

He told me that last Friday's ultrasound revealed that the fluid buildup in my liver is now gone, which is the reason my abdomen no longer seems to be as swollen. A quick physical exam confirmed this. My abdomen is no longer hard, one side of my liver is normal, and the other is much less swollen than it was. He called it a "dramatic improvement."

What the ultrasound did not reveal was any sign that my tumours are shrinking. I do feel a bit disappointed, but it is early days yet, and all other signs show that the treatment is working.

I'm pleased.

For the moment, the forces of good seem to have the upper hand.

The Bell

Sometime between my last go-round with chemo (the one that ended in the summer, prior to radiation and the recurrence) and my latest diagnosis, a bell was installed in the chemo room.

It's pretty nifty. When someone completes his or her last chemotherapy treatment, he or she rings the bell on the way out and everyone claps. It's a wonderful idea. I remember feeling after my last treatment in June that I would have liked there to be some way to mark the end and my survival.

Hearing the bell ring during my treatment on Tuesday made me happy, but also a bit sad. There is unlikely to be a time when I will get to ring that bell—no triumphant moment when the cancer is behind me. My treatments will go on indefinitely and, even when I take breaks, there will likely always be more chemo on the horizon.

I've more or less come to terms with this, and the chemo regimen I'm on is so much gentler than my first experience, especially now that the Herceptin side effects are under control.

I really did get through the first go-round by counting down the cycles, and marking each with a present to myself! And I did feel triumphant when I finished, even without a bell to ring.

I still do. That first round of chemo was really hard. Having cancer is hard, but I'm doing okay. Much of the time I feel quite content, even happy. All in all, I think that I'm handling things really well.

Groundhog Day, Revisited

It was a year ago today that I had my mastectomy. The memories are still very fresh.

I remember my anxiety turning to raw terror as I lay in the operating room. I could see the surgical tools and hear them clink as they were readied for surgery.

I remember the anaesthesiologist's soothing voice, and that he asked me about my children in order to get me to relax. This worked much better than when he asked me about work. I don't remember falling asleep.

I remember the euphoria of waking, knowing that it was over. And I remember the whole host of emotions as I rode the roller coaster to recovery. I still ride that roller coaster, only now the hills are a little less steep.

I felt sad today, grieving not just for my lost breast, but for all the ways in which cancer has ravaged my body. Menopause at thirty-eight, thinning hair and eyebrows, and, yes, the ridge of scar that runs from the centre of my chest to my shoulder, not to mention the loss of mobility brought on by radiation. My face and body have been irrevocably changed by cancer. I gave myself permission to be a little bit sad today.

What Price Peace?

Today was a chemo day (just chemo, no Herceptin), so I have, of course, spent the evening in bed feeling yucky.

From the upstairs bedroom, I overheard the following, which took place on the ground floor of our house:

DANIEL: "I want to watch *Scooby Doo Meets Batman* now." (Incidentally, this is probably one of the worst videos of all time.)

TIM: "It's dinnertime. You can watch some of the video after you've eaten. Come to the table now."

DANIEL: "I want to watch *Scooby Doo* NOW!!!"

TIM: "Daniel, you have two choices. You can watch the video after you've eaten your dinner or you can go to your room."

[Insert increasingly hysterical repetitions of "I want to watch the video now," until they have crescendoed into a full-fledged tantrum.]

SACHA: "Daniel, if you stop crying, I'll give you a penny."

DANIEL: "Okay."

Daniel went to the table and ate his dinner happily. When he was done, Sacha gave him a penny.

My spouse and I are fully cognizant of the myriad ways in which this was problematic, but we did think the whole thing was pretty funny. And Sacha did get his brother to eat.

On Being Afraid

Sometimes,
it clutches at my heart
icy fingers squeezing
so hard I cannot breathe.

Sometimes,
it whispers in my ear
quiet murmurs disquiet
as I go about life's tasks.

Sometimes,
I am ambushed
sucker-punched
when I have let down my guard.

Like all intimate relationships
ours ebbs and flows in its intensity
but we never part for long.

I live with fear
but not in fear.

And I will never let fear rule my life.

In My Bones, or "There Is No Stage 5"

The thing about living with stage 4 breast cancer is that every change in how my body functions can feel suspicious. After all, feeling a stitch in my side led to a diagnosis of metastasis, so when I experienced bloating and relatively mild abdominal pain this week, I began to feel a bit concerned.

Actually, that is a gross understatement; before yesterday's appointment with my oncologist, I was completely beside myself with pure terror.

You see, I've been feeling good—really good. And what happened the last couple of times I felt this good? I found a lump in my breast. I found out that the cancer had spread to my liver, so I became certain that I was going to be told that my prognosis had just dramatically worsened.

But my oncologist was, in his way, very reassuring. He told me that he was pretty certain that what I have been experiencing is "nothing," and he confirmed this when he examined me. He doesn't think that my liver is any more swollen than it was a couple of weeks ago. He did, however, order another ultrasound just in case.

As for my fear of spreading, well, he said that I shouldn't worry because it is a certainty that the cancer has spread to other parts of my body. As he put it, cancer cells are not selective about where they go, so I shouldn't worry about it spreading to my other organs and my bones because, well, it's already there.

He said I should think of my cancer as a chronic illness that we will work at managing with various therapies, and that when one stops working, we will try something else. He also said he was much less worried about me than he was in November: "It's a cause for concern when a patient turns yellow."

As I write this, I am pink from the cold and feeling more relaxed than I have in days. Once again, I am reminded of how much fighting this illness is about staying strong emotionally, as well as physically.

Business Ventures

Sacha and I had the following conversation as our dog Jasper and I walked him to school the other day:

SACHA: "I have an idea for an Internet venture for dogs. I'd call it 'iSmell.' The website would describe a whole list of smells and you could choose the one you think your dog would like best and order a patch with that smell."

ME: "That's a great idea! But the smells would have to be pretty disgusting."

SACHA: "The more disgusting, the more expensive."

ME: "Old socks, rotting meat ..."

SACHA: "Exactly. We could have a page listing all the newest smells and the home page would have a list of the top-selling smells."

ME: "That reminds me, Papa tells me that you were making a vending machine when you were supposed to be in bed last night."

SACHA: "Yeah. And it works, too, except no one wants to buy my product."

ME: "Why not?"

SACHA: "Because it costs a dollar and the product is a penny."

Sunday, February 25, 2007

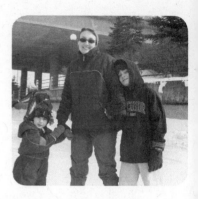

Channelling Peggy Lee

"Is that all there is, is that all there is?
If that's all there is, my friends, then
let's keep dancing ..."

I am tolerating chemo relatively well. I am no longer experiencing the roller coaster of Herceptin's side effects, but the routine is grinding me down: Two weeks on, one week off. And there is no end in sight, at least not an end I want to spend much time thinking about.

When I am feeling well, and even much of the time when I am not, I am rarely bored. I am, however, struggling to fight some serious malaise. Not that long ago, life felt full of possibility. There were paths to choose and decisions to be made, and if any particular path didn't please me, I could easily change direction and try a new one.

Now that I am not working outside the home (my oncologist says that no insurance company would ever expect me to work again), I have time for other creative pursuits, but I need to shake off the funk brought on by two weeks on, one week off.

I just have to keep putting one foot in front of the other. Today, I am going to do that in a pair of skates. Despite living three minutes (on foot) from the canal, I haven't skated in a couple of years.

"If that's all there is, my friends, then let's keep dancing."

Words to Live by

Sometimes the fear and sadness really do come from out of nowhere. Yesterday I was sitting and knitting, waiting for my boys to finish swimming lessons. As I looked up to see my youngest running toward me, the thought hit me: *I won't be around when he starts high school.* The thought quite literally knocked the wind out of me. I pushed it away and we went on with our evening. The sadness did linger, though.

Then today, as I unpacked a bag of goodies given to me at a very belated birthday dinner (remember that my birthday was August 4), I pulled out, among many other lovely things, a mug with the following on it: "Life is not measured by the number of breaths we take but by the moments that take our breath away." (Anonymous)

That pretty much sums up my approach to life these days. I have a friend who often refers to "living on borrowed time." We all live on borrowed time. What matters is making that time count. I'm trying to do that.

The same wonderful women who gave me the mug also gave me a card that says, "Between me and insanity stand my friends." Amen to that.

I may outlive the doctor's predictions, and am doing what I can to make that happen, but I am also trying to enjoy the present and to savour those moments that take my breath away.

I Am Awesome

I walk through the snow, pushing a stroller filled with preschooler, library books, and a birthday cake. I walk the dog on a day when wind brings tears to my eyes that freeze on my eyelashes. I walk long and hard, my heart pumping. My legs are strong and muscular. My face glows with exertion. I am fit and healthy. When I walk, I am not a cancer patient.

Skin Deep

Yesterday, when we were sitting in the hospital waiting room, Tim stroked my face and said, "Wrinkles." I cringed, but he meant it as a good thing.

He tells me that I am more beautiful as I get older and he loves every line on my face.

Since he has always found me the most attractive when I am dressed casually and looking relaxed (the man thinks overalls are hot), I believe him. The "eye of the beholder," indeed.

Raging

I am feeling seriously pissed off tonight. I am angry that I have cancer, fed up with my lymphedema, and furious at the lousy prognosis associated with liver metastases.

In the comments at one of my favourite blogs, "d.i.y./not d-i-e" (now, unfortunately, off-line), Rebel1in8* writes: "Part of empowering someone with cancer is allowing them the right to bitch without the fear that they are sending out a message of defeat and whining."

Exactly. I am still a "glass half full" sort of person, but tonight, the water in the glass is boiling.

*http://rebel1in8.blogspot.com

■ Saturday, March 31, 2007

Model Mom

Anecdote 1

The doorbell rang at about noon today. My youngest son and I were still in our pyjamas. I answered to find a smiling woman with a bible under her arm and a religious leaflet in her hand. Before she could launch into her spiel, I firmly but politely said, "We're not interested," and closed the door.

I turned around to find my not-quite-four-year-old standing with his pants around his ankles and a big smile on his face. "I'm showing my penis," he said proudly. We immediately had a conversation about private body parts.

I do wonder what exactly the lady at the door had time to see and what horrified thoughts crossed her mind.

Anecdote 2

My older son had the day off from school yesterday. We went out for a short walk to a nearby store. Inside, one of the clerks was admiring our dog. "I think he would like me to pet him," she said.

"Go ahead, he smells better than he sometimes does," said my not-quite-nine-year-old. "He hasn't had a bath in a year. My longest stretch was from September until last week," he boasted.

I was back in the same store today, this time with just the dog. The store was very crowded and a number of people were lined up behind me at the cash. "I remember you," said the clerk. "I thought it was funny when your son said he hadn't bathed in seven months." It's those little moments that make a mother proud.

New Kind of Cycle

So maybe I don't get PMS anymore, but my moods are as tied to a cycle as they've ever been. My heart is lighter today and the sadness and fear I've been feeling seem to have evaporated.

I do not have chemo next week.

And that makes everything better.

More Than the Sum of My Parts

A liver riddled with tumours.

A scar where my right breast used to be.

Lymphedema in my back and arm.

Frozen shoulder from radiation.

Radiation burns on my chest and back.

Assorted minor but annoying side effects from chemotherapy.

Fifteen pounds gained in 2007.

Panic every time I feel a stitch in my right side.

Some days it feels relentless. I start to fix one problem only to be plagued with another.

And it doesn't help that very few health care practitioners actually seem to see me as a whole person.

Life and Death

I have a stitch in my right side tonight. It's probably nothing, but since my liver functions are also a little elevated, my doctor is ordering another ultrasound. Suddenly, "stable" (the condition of my tumours as of my last CT scan) is looking pretty good.

I try not to dwell on my fears. There are, however, times when the dark thoughts that nibble at the edge of my consciousness threaten to swallow me whole.

I want to live longer than the friend of a friend (and mother of young children), who died from liver mets within two years of her diagnosis. I want to outlive the prognosis of "years, not decades" that was gently delivered by my oncologist. I want to be a living, breathing medical miracle.

I want to live.

■ **Wednesday, April 18, 2007**

So Damned Tired

I am bordering on neutropenic again, which could explain why I have been feeling so rundown. My white blood count was very low on Tuesday, not low enough to cancel chemo, but getting there.

I have an ultrasound scheduled for April 30, and will get results at an appointment on May 4. Meanwhile, I know the following:

- My liver is swollen, but not terribly so and nowhere near where it was in November.

- My liver functions in two of the categories they test are normal. A third area was high, but it is also the one the doctors worry about the least as it can be indicative of other things going on with the body.

- It is not a good sign that I have been experiencing discomfort, but my most constant stitch is nowhere near my liver. I really need to learn more about my own anatomy.

- The swelling and the fatigue could also be the result of my battered immune system.

I am feeling less stressed than I was on the weekend, which isn't saying much, given that I was a wreck on the weekend, and reassured enough that my worries are no longer top of mind, so keep your fingers crossed for me.

And stay away from me if you are sick. And for goodness sake, wash your hands after you go to the bathroom. (This is for the guy

Tim almost confronted at the cancer centre today, and who I'm sure isn't reading this.)

■ **Friday, April 20, 2007**

Ending Better Than It Started

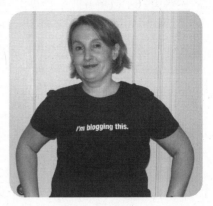

Monday

Found out someone used my credit card number and forged my signature on a Visa cheque for almost $2,000. The cheque was returned as NSF. Fortunately, we've been spending beyond our means or the fraud might have been successful. As it is, we've had to cancel our credit card and wait for a new one to be sent to us.

Tuesday

Chemo.

Wednesday

Appointment with my radiation oncologist. I was first examined by a medical student, who asked, sounding alarmed, "How long have you had this lump?" I panicked for a moment, then realized she was referring to my portacath. Shouldn't she have known what it was?

As for the doctor, should a man who is uncomfortable with the words "bra" and "prosthesis" really be working as a radiation oncologist with breast cancer patients? He seemed disbelieving when I told him that the treated area on my chest and back is still extremely tender and had no suggestions as to what I could do to ease this discomfort. When I told him that it hurts too much to wear a prosthesis, he said, "Well, you have to wear something in public."

This is the same doctor who objected to the fact that I do not have the same last name as my spouse.

Thankfully, this same spouse was once again in attendance. It was one of those appointments when it was really good to have someone there who knows me well, if only to say afterwards, "You are not crazy."

Tim has decided that I need to get a T-shirt that says "I'm blogging this" and wear it to all future appointments. I think he's right.

Thursday
Booked my plane ticket to Chicago to attend BlogHer '07, a women's blogging conference, thanks to air miles donated by my wonderful brother-in-law.

Nothing contributes to a sense of optimism like making plans a few months in advance. And just thinking about spending a weekend with other women bloggers makes my heart beat a little faster.

Friday
Spring has sprung. I feel quite a bit better. And I finished the little blanket that grew, my "log cabin" from Mason-Dixon Knitting. Knitting an almost queen-sized blanket does give one a sense of accomplishment. It is the most beautiful thing that I have ever made and it makes me happy just to look at it. It's been almost finished for weeks since our return from our road trip to Florida, where I worked on it in the car, both ways. And it smells good too, since I washed the potato chip smell out of it this afternoon. (Did I mention that I worked on it on a long car trip?)

Things are definitely looking up.

Sieve

Today, I went to an appointment with my naturopath. I was early.
Three days early.

Chemo is eating my brain.

■ **Tuesday, April 24, 2007**

Whiskers on Kittens

I came up with this list this morning:

- runners' legs

- dog snoring

- my coffee mug

- the smell of lilacs

- sunflowers

- dark chocolate dipped in coffee

- soft, beautiful yarn made from natural fibres

- Greg Brown's voice

- the back of my sons' necks

Heartbreaker

An older woman (she was at least six) said to my four-year-old son, this evening, "You've stolen my heart."

They had known each other for approximately twenty minutes, and met while we waited for a big enough table to be ready at a restaurant. She was the manager's daughter and they had been chasing each other around the restaurant foyer.

After we were seated, she came to our table and said, "I wish I could sit beside him."

This kind of thing happens everywhere we go with Daniel. I shudder to think what the future brings. Let's just hope he uses his charisma wisely.

$150,000

That is how much it costs to treat a woman with Herceptin for a year. Drug companies are evil. Thank goodness, once again, for socialized medicine. And, boy, it costs a lot to keep me alive.

Covered in Slime

I hate ultrasounds. It's not just the unpleasantness of lying in a chilly room, covered in cold, goopy gel.

It's not just the ugly robe and mind-numbing boredom of lying first on my back and then my sides as I silently obey commands to "Breathe in. Hold it. Breathe out."

What really gets to me is the fact that there is a screen right in front of me that I cannot interpret, a screen that has the answers to whether the tumours in my liver have grown larger, or if they have started to invade elsewhere.

I hate that the ultrasound technician, a stranger, can interpret the images yet can tell me nothing. I really hate ultrasounds.

I see the oncologist on Friday. I hope to have results by then.

Once Burned

I have been trying very hard to think positively this week. This was greatly helped by my naturopath, who walked me through a terrific relaxation exercise. And for the rest of this week, I have been dutifully repeating, "Every day and in every way, I am getting better and better," along with the more cumbersome, "Negative thoughts and negative feelings do not influence me at any level of my mind." And it's been working—until today.

Today I heard that insistent voice that started as a whisper and built to a roar—the voice that reminds me that I was pretty damn positive when I first went through treatment and before I knew that the cancer had metastasized. A fat lot of good it did me then, but it is not helpful to imagine my tumours growing, imagine myself sick from a more toxic chemo regimen, imagine myself dying, or to imagine trying to explain to my children that Mama is dying. Not helpful at all.

Mind you, I do believe in the value of a good meltdown. I wish tears came to me more easily, but dwelling on the unthinkable does not help me cope with stress, and there is some evidence that positive thought can actually help with healing. So ... all together now: "Every day and in every way, I am getting better and better."

Ultrasound results tomorrow.

"Grossly Stable"

To paraphrase my ultrasound report, I still have extensive metastasis, but my condition is "essentially grossly unchanged." My other organs are "unremarkable." There is no fluid buildup.

"IMPRESSION: Grossly stable liver disease."

Jeez, do you think the radiologist could have qualified her opinions any more? ("Please note that it is extremely difficult to accurately compare between two ultrasound studies.")

I'll take it, though.

My liver functions are pretty close to normal again, too. So ... I still don't know what is causing the stitch, but it's not bigger tumours eating my liver.

My doctor, who works with my oncologist, is going to order another CT scan, which can provide a more detailed analysis, but doesn't feel that this needs to be done urgently. It will be ordered for a couple of months from now as part of regular testing and in lieu of my next ultrasound. That reassured me as much as anything.

I am very relieved.

A Song by Daniel

I love my Mama
And she is so beautiful.
But she doesn't read me comic books
She reads me books.

I love my Papa, too.
And he reads me comic books
And he reads me books.

I Don't Have Cancer

Daniel and I left the house at 1:30 this afternoon. He rode in the stroller and I pushed him.

We were bound for the library, but as he announced that he was taking a nap, I took the long way and walked for an hour along the canal.

We chose movies and books at the library and then went for pizza slices. I read to him while we ate.

We then moved on to our local fair-trade coffee shop for iced green tea with mint (me) and chocolate milk (him). We read more books on the patio.

Then it was time to make stops for dog treats for the dog and a new toothbrush for Daniel.

When our errands were done, we went to the park, where I chased him around for a while and then chatted with a couple of other moms I know while he played.

Then we went home for dinner. We had been out for four and a half hours.

After dinner I washed Daniel's hair, despite his howls of protest, and then sat with him as he played in the bath. Finally, I dried him off, got him ready for bed, read him two stories, and kissed him goodnight.

Does this sound like a day in the life of a cancer patient? Not to me it doesn't.

Dos and Don'ts for Health Care Professionals

- Do introduce yourself. I once had a doctor come into a room and start writing on my chest without speaking to me.

- Don't look horrified when I tell you I have metastatic breast cancer.

- Do ask my permission before turning my test/appointment/ treatment into a lesson for a student.

- Don't talk about me as though I am not in the room.

- Don't ask me questions about my treatment that are irrelevant to the procedure being performed and/or outside your sphere of knowledge.

- Don't tell me about your aunt/friend/cousin who was unsuccessfully treated for cancer.

- Don't tell me that the above-mentioned aunt/friend/cousin was unsuccessfully treated with one of the drugs I have told you has been part of my regimen.

- Do thank me for my patience, especially if the test/treatment/ procedure took twice as long as it normally would because you are still learning how to do it.

What If?

A story on the news last night really threw me for a loop. It seems that regular consumption of vitamin D can reduce the risk of cancer by as much as 60 percent. Hearing that made me feel quite sick, actually. I know that prevention is not a simple thing, but I can't help asking, "What if?"

Nine-Year-Old Boys

I am alone in the house with two very excited pre-pubescent boys right now. They are both lovely people, brilliant, quirky, and enormously entertaining. I was privy to the following conversation on our walk home:

NOAH (MY SON'S FRIEND): "I'm trying to grow a goatee. (Strokes his chin and thrusts it forward) How am I doing?"

SACHA: "I'm growing a ponytail. It's been a really long time since I had a haircut. My hair is so long I need to brush it almost every day and wash it once a week."

Honestly, I have to remind this child several times to use soap when he bathes, and he still doesn't always remember.

I can't wait to see what these kids are like as teenagers.

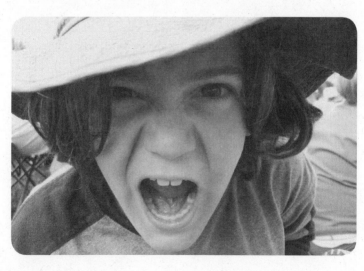

Of Neutrophils and Liver Functions

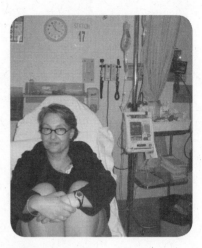

I had chemo and Herceptin yesterday. I always drag my ass to the first treatment after my week off. It's especially hard to go into treatment when I've had a few days to feel like myself. My head is still fuzzy from the Demerol I take to mitigate the side effects from the Herceptin, but, all in all, I could be feeling worse.

I had blood work done yesterday, as I always do before chemo. I have become obsessed with the results. Yesterday's results were interesting.

My neutrophils (the white blood cells that fight infection) were very low. They were so low, in fact, that if they had been any lower, chemo would have been cancelled. This also helps explain why I have been feeling so tired. The trick over the next week will be to remember my Neupogen injections (all five of them), to wash my hands (and my kids' hands) a lot, and to stay away from sick people.

Additionally and more importantly, all my liver functions were well within the range of normal for the first time in many months. I am very pleased about this. I choose to believe that this is a sign that my upcoming CT scan (scheduled for next week) will bring good news as well. Perhaps even news of shrinking tumours?

Of course, another report that all is stable would be good, but I'm in the mood to indulge in a little wild optimism.

No Deconstruction Needed

I have just started another knitting project. It's another giant under-
taking, even bigger than the giant log-cabin blanket I finished in
March because I will have to sew pieces together. I don't think I need
a psychologist to tell me why I am drawn to projects that will take
me a really long time to finish. I am, after all, an optimist at heart.

■ **Saturday, June 23, 2007**

And the Rain Came down

Last Friday night, I had a meltdown. I can count on one hand the number of times I have cried since being diagnosed with breast cancer in late 2005.

I cried a couple of weeks after my surgery, a response to fear, frustration, and grief.

I cried when my beloved dog died.

And I probably cried when I found out about the metastasis, but my memory of that time is clouded by shock, pain, and the drugs used to numb it all.

Other than that, there have been a few teary moments, but no honest-to-goodness meltdowns. I was due.

It was a conversation with Tim that set me off. It wasn't his fault. He merely expressed reservations about a proposed getaway. Every insecurity I have ever felt about being lovable came to the surface, as well as the emotional toll of how cancer has changed my body. I felt rejected, and I dissolved into a sobbing, gasping puddle. But really, I'd been primed for a meltdown for days.

I had had a very busy week as I usually do on my weeks off from chemo. By Thursday, when I went to see my physiotherapist, I was running on fumes. She made a casual comment about an aunt who had liver mets, and who'd had a wonderful active life, post-diagnosis. She added, "And she lived another eight or nine years."

I am not yet forty years old. In eight years, my youngest son will be only twelve. I will be lucky to live another eight years, and I will likely be in treatment right until the end.

She intended her words as a kindness, but they hit me hard. I didn't respond or even dwell much on her comment, but it stayed inside me. I was cranky with my naturopath and out of sorts for the next twenty-four hours.

Tension built, the clouds broke, and then down came the rain. Like all good summer storms, though, the air felt lighter after it ended. The sky was a little bluer this week and the sun shone brightly. My step has been a little lighter, too, even with a chemo treatment.

And can I say how lucky I am to live with a man who knows what to do in a meltdown, understands why they're necessary, and never expects either apology or explanation? He's even come around on the getaway plans.

I Feel Like Celebrating

I was very, very tired this morning and went back to bed instead of going to yoga. We'd had a lovely but busy weekend and I woke up exhausted.

I was feeling a little guilty about hanging around in my pyjamas until my friend Deb asked me what I'd done this weekend. Before I'd finished the list, I realized exactly why it was that I was so tired: Sacha had two friends over for a twenty-four-hour play date; I walked with Daniel to the library; went out to lunch, and then to soccer; on Sunday, we went to the market; I had a physio appointment; we took the kids to the park; and then Sacha and I went for a walk.

I gave myself permission to stay in my pyjamas until late in the afternoon. I was in a very good mood this evening. Tim took Daniel out to hear some jazz and my friend Helen came over with her new dog. We walked Sacha over to his friend's house (yes, I know it's a school night, but it's almost the end of the year and the boys wanted to watch *Doctor Who* together), and then strolled a bit before heading back to my house. It was then that I realized that I felt like celebrating.

We had local strawberries with whipped cream and a bottle of ice wine we'd saved from our trip last fall to Niagara-on-the-Lake. We drank the wine in champagne flutes because that's what you do when you celebrate.

It is only now, as I sit at the computer, that I stop to articulate my reasons for celebrating, and I realize that I have too many to count.

My lovely neighbourhood.

My dog's joy in going for a walk.

Sacha's pride as he held the leash, directed us to his friend's house, and greeted the kids he knew along the way.

The way both my sons light up when they see me.

Friends and family who love me.

The fact that I am alive, pain-free, and able to go for a walk with a dear friend on a hot summer evening.

And aren't fresh strawberries and whipped cream a good reason to celebrate in their own right?

Off to the Spa

The month-long birthday extravaganza begins today (I am turning forty on August 4). I am off to the spa with my friend Deb. We will get facials and pedicures, drink lots of wine, and watch a movie in our pyjamas. Deb is the only friend I trust to share a bed with me and not make fun of me for snoring.

Also, Daniel started at the daycare in his new school today (he starts JK in the fall). To say that he was eager and ready is an understatement. On the way over he made us practise our lines: "You say, 'Have a good day, son.'"

I think my children may watch too much television.

Part Four

The New Normal

Holy Shit!

I learned the results from my CT scan today: "There has been very substantial response to treatment. Widespread metastatic disease to the liver has regressed remarkably.... Very significant response to chemotherapy ... the remaining parenchymal nodules and evidence of scarring are difficult to evaluate for viable residual disease." In other words, they could find no evidence of the cancer, just scars to show where the tumours once were.

The doctor who works with my oncologist said, as she passed me the report, "I want to frame this." She was beaming.

This doesn't mean I can quit chemo or especially Herceptin, but it does mean that at least over the summer, I will go less frequently, receiving treatment every three weeks. There are very likely still cancer cells in my body, but they appear to be impossible to locate at the moment.

As my doctor said, "This is as good as it gets."

I am in shock, and completely elated. I keep rereading my CT scan report and have yet to bring myself to tell anyone. (Tim knows because he was with me.) I was very optimistic that I would at least learn that my tumours were stable and was hoping for even better news. But this, honestly, is almost beyond my wildest dreams.

Going to go pinch myself now.

Dear Friends: You Overwhelm Me

I am overwhelmed by all the good wishes I have received via every possible media in the last couple of days.

After the initial rush of joy at learning my good news, I admit to being numb for the next twenty-four hours or so. I couldn't quite believe that the tumours could be gone. It was also really weird to be shocked by good news for a change, but the shock has worn off and now I am positively giddy.

And it gets better. My wonderful friends have given me the most amazing birthday present. I was presented today with a cheque that will completely cover all of my BlogHer expenses and then some—all of them except for air travel, which is covered by points from my brother-in-law.

I knew that some money was coming (a couple of people had let this slip). I knew that my friends were making it possible for me to go to Chicago, but I am completely and utterly overwhelmed by their generosity. I don't have the words to express my gratitude. I am even a little embarrassed, and very, very touched.

Planning for BlogHer has been very important. The mere act of making a commitment to attend something several months ahead of time felt like a defiance of cancer. I had to plan on being healthy and fit because I had committed to this trip. The very idea got me through some difficult days and nights.

I have the best friends in the world.

Cancelled

Chemo was cancelled due to low neutrophils (the white blood cells that fight infection) today. I went in by myself for the first time, which was fine, thanks to a borrowed CD player and a talking book, and was, frankly, shocked when they sent me home. They won't administer chemotherapy if neutrophils dip below 1.0. Mine were at 0.8, and they didn't bother with Herceptin since I have to go back for chemo anyway.

But now I'm feeling pretty rundown and my throat is scratchy. I took the dog out for a walk and couldn't go for more than a few blocks. I am wiped out.

Is it the power of suggestion or am I really rundown? I'll find out tomorrow when I go back to the cancer centre, get blood work done again, wait for the results, and then either go home or get treated.

I'm hoping I get treated since the rest of the summer has been pretty much plotted out. The kids are in camp when they need to be, off when I will be feeling well, and we have planned a couple of getaways, including the trip to Chicago.

I have plans, dammit.

Treated and Home

And stoned. My counts were just high enough today to go ahead. As usual, the Demerol-Gravol cocktail made me very stoned very fast. I think it's very amusing for anyone with me, including the oncology nurses.

I fell asleep during treatment, came home, and slept for four and a half more hours.

I am still stoned, but happy that I don't need to go back until July 31.

■ **Monday, July 16, 2007**

Faces

I love this pic, with my face and my son's in profile and our friend
in the painting looking over our shoulders. I also love how shaggy
my hair looks. I have hair! And new specs. I love the relationship
captured in this moment. And I love how healthy I look.

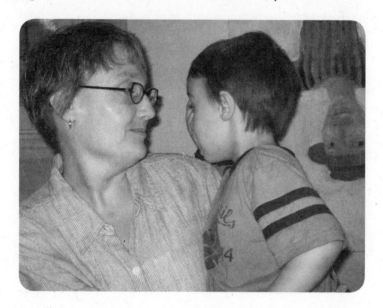

Anxious

I've been feeling a low-level anxiety for the last few days. I'm not sure if I am unsure about my future, waiting for the other shoe to drop, or simply stressed that my sweetie's passport has not yet arrived in advance of our trip to Chicago.

Last night I felt stuck in a loop. I can't remember the dream I had, but I kept waking up in a panic, calming myself down, and then having the same dream again. I woke up exhausted.

This afternoon, I was distracted by the antics of two nine-year-old boys. ("Please close the door before the cat gets out. Please close the door. Indoor voices, please. I don't want to talk about vomit. Please don't talk with your mouth full. Stop spraying the cat with the water bottle. I really don't want to talk about vomit. No, you can't play with the paper shredder. I will give you ice cream if you go eat it outside and leave me alone.") This evening, the funny feeling returned to the pit of my stomach.

It helped to knit in front of the television tonight, although please remind me never to watch "Law and Order: Special Victims Unit" again, no matter how desperate I am. I find the process of knitting very soothing. My mitred squares are perfect and relaxing. Each little square is a satisfying project unto itself. If I never get around to sewing, I'll have 120 beautiful pot holders.

And now I am off to bed (much too late). I am hoping for a dreamless and uninterrupted sleep.

Milestone

My baby packed his bag and hit the road today. Sacha, at age nine, ready for a play date and sleepover at his friend's house, packed his own overnight gear with some prompting from me—"Toothbrush? Underwear? Stuffed animals?"—stuck his helmet on his head, hopped on his bike, and rode off.

"Bye! See you tomorrow!"

He was adamant that I not accompany him. I told him to call when he got there. I rushed into the house and called his friend. "Sacha is on his way. Make sure he phones me as soon as he arrives." Five minutes later, he did. It was only six blocks, after all. He was fine. I, on the other hand, am a little traumatized.

■ **Tuesday, July 24, 2007**

10 Seconds for BlogHer

This was the introduction I wrote for the slide show that was part of the BlogHer welcome session:

> My friends gave me this trip to Chicago as a fortieth birthday present.
>
> My birthday is on August 4.
>
> I am a full-time cancer patient, living a really full life.
>
> I have been with my spouse for more than sixteen years.
>
> It was *not* love at first sight.
>
> I must not have been wearing my glasses.
>
> My sons are as different as two boys can be, except that they are both brilliant, beautiful, and loving.
>
> They also drive me crazy and I love them beyond all measure.
>
> I love Scrabble, wine, dark chocolate, knitting, and a really good book.
>
> I love the way my dog smells.
>
> I am completely bilingual in French and English.
>
> I am happy.
>
> This was more than ten seconds.

Women Like Me

A poem for a hot day:

Voyeur
Women's breasts emerge in the heat of the summer.
Big ones and small ones.
Perky ones (I could fit them in my hand).
Breasts nursing babies.
Freckled cleavage.
Wrinkled cleavage.
And breasts that can't possibly be real.
I stare at women's breasts now with great fascination.
And not a little envy.
I have never seen a woman with one breast.
Except in the mirror.

He Cracks Me up

Daniel, in the bath, playing with his knight and castle bath toys: "This knight just got killed." We got these in Chicago and used them to bribe him to wash his hair. Not sure how to top this; we may have to resort to offering him cash.

TIM: "I don't like killing."

DANIEL: "He didn't get killed. He died because he was old, and an arrow went through him."

Observation 1: At least he knows what his parents' values are even if he hasn't completely absorbed them.

Observation 2: That Y chromosome has a pretty strong influence. Parenthood has made me renounce long-held convictions in the nature-nurture debate.

Bittersweet Milestone

In an hour, I will be forty. The celebrating began in early July and I have been very, very spoiled.

Life is good and I have more reason for hope than I have had in a long time. But I would be lying if I did not admit that this birthday is a bit tinged with sadness.

My life, at forty, does not look the way I thought it would. Cancer has irrevocably changed me and the choices I will make. My expectations and aspirations will never again be what they once were, so, yes, I'm a little sad, but I have, thus far, defied medical expectations and I am determined that I will continue to do so.

I have a beautiful family and a community of friends who have, in turn, exceeded my expectations of love and friendship. I am feeling more creative, inspired, and confident than I have since childhood, and it feels like more good things are just around the corner.

I need to indulge this sadness, to give it voice, and as I write, it dissipates.

Tomorrow, we head to the family cottage, one of my favourite places in the world, where I will be reunited with Sacha, whom I have not seen in almost two weeks (he has been hanging out with his cousins). I have missed him more than he has missed me, which is as it should be, and I can't wait to hug him.

I think I am going to have a very good birthday, and it's going to be a good year. I can feel it.

So This Is What It Looks Like

I had my regular pre-chemo appointment with my oncologist yesterday. Having had time to get over the wonderful shock of my CT scan results, I had a few questions:

Q: Can my chemo schedule be scaled back now?

A: Yes!

.I pause to do a few cartwheels, at least in my head. Instead of a week of Herceptin and Vinorelbine, a week of just vino and then one week off, I will have two weeks of treatment and then two weeks off. Is this about as clear as mud? Another way to put it is that instead of being in treatment two-thirds of the time, I'll be in treatment only half the time, although this exaggerates the impact because I always have treatment on Tuesdays and feel better by the weekend.

Q: So, what are we treating now since there don't appear to be any tumours on my liver?

A: Once you are in stage 4, you assume that the cancer is systemic and you need to treat it head to toe with a systemic drug.

My oncologist actually said that at this stage, they could give me lethal doses of chemo, followed by a bone marrow transplant, and still find cancer somewhere in my body. If my cancer was the kind that responds to hormonal treatments (and referred to as hormone-positive or estrogen/progesterone-positive), I would have had more options available to me. Hormone-positive breast cancers are also generally considered to be less aggressive and more responsive to treatment, including treatment in pill form, such as Tamoxifen or the newer aromatase inhibitors. However, the only treatments currently available to me are intravenous, specifically Herceptin and chemotherapy.

Q: But things are looking much more hopeful than they were last November? (Asked very tentatively)

A: An emphatic yes. I should expect, however, that I will need to change my treatment at some point when this one stops working. He did make it very clear, though, that he has many other options in his arsenal.

Q: Should we credit the Herceptin for the dramatic improvement in my condition?

A: Vinorelbine and Herceptin have been shown to work remarkably well in combination with each other, but, yes, Herceptin is a wonderful drug. I am very fortunate that my cancer surfaced after it was approved in Canada for treatment of breast cancer.

Q: Is this what it means to be in remission?

A: Yes, it does.

So there you have it. I'll have a bit of non-chemo time in the next little while and I have a lot more reason for hope. Not so long ago, daring to hope to attend the BlogHer conference seemed like hubris. Now I'm working on a couple of big projects and doing a little planning for the future. It feels good.

The Hardest

I wrote last year, after finishing chemo (the first six rounds, which were supposed to cure me), that it was the hardest thing I'd ever done. But yesterday, I was reminded that I was wrong.

The hardest thing that I have ever done was tell my oldest son that I have cancer. And then that it had come back. To knowingly inflict pain this way on my child ... I don't really have the words to express how much this hurt.

"Blondie" and I met at the BlogHer conference. We had a conversation at the end of a wine-soaked evening during which she told me about her mother's cancer. Blondie told me how she would sneak into her mother's room and hold a mirror under her mouth, just to make sure she was still breathing. The very thought makes me gasp a little.

Like Blondie's mom, who is now healthy, I spent the days following each chemo, which were always over a weekend, lying in the dark, unable to tolerate movement, sound, or light. My spouse, as well as family and friends, would make sure these weekends were full of distractions for the boys, but I know they found it confusing and frightening that their mother was unable to respond to their needs.

And then, last fall, I put chemo and radiation behind me and returned to work, only to find out within weeks that the cancer had spread to my liver. When the oncologist confirmed this diagnosis, you'll recall that my first words were, "I have two beautiful children!"

When we told Sacha, who was then only eight years old, about the recurrence, he was very stoic and calm. We explained that I would once again be in treatment, but that I had very good doctors and that we were going to do everything we could to fight the cancer. This time, he didn't ask if I was going to die. I'm glad because I didn't want to lie to him.

I was in so much pain during that time and so swollen from fluid buildup on my liver. Those first few weeks after the metastasis was diagnosed are very blurred in my memory, made hazy by shock, pain, and the drugs used to relieve those things. And through it all, Sacha did not talk about the cancer. Then one day, after the dust had settled and the benefits of much gentler chemo had begun to take effect, there was an incident at school that revealed how much anxiety he'd been bottling up inside.

I took him home, and told him that the principal had told me what happened. I told him that I wasn't angry. I said that I loved him very much and that he could talk to me about anything. I told him that I was already feeling much better, which was true, and that I wasn't going anywhere any time soon. And I set about finding a therapist.

But Sacha balked at the idea of talking to a therapist. As the weeks and then months passed and my health was obviously improving (and ultrasounds indicated that the tumours had stabilized), we saw him relax. By the time we went to Florida in March, he was the happiest, most confident, and most at ease that he had been, not just since the cancer, but since starting school a couple of years previously.

He ended up having a great year at school and in July, we were able to share the good news with him about what my latest CT scan had revealed. The therapist got put on the back-burner. But a post that Blondie wrote on her own blog* has me thinking that it might be time to make finding a therapist a priority—someone Sacha could meet and to whom he could turn should he need to talk, because who knows what the future will bring? I plan to continue to defy expectations, but I need to make sure that my children are cared for in every way, and no matter what. I realize, too, that the impact of cancer could manifest itself months, years, or even decades into the future. Even little Daniel, who seems oblivious (but who knows how much he is taking in?), will not remember a time when his mother did not have cancer.

I've done a lot of work in therapy dealing with issues from my own childhood. As Blondie writes, *"My particular Childhood Thing happens to be cancer, but if it hadn't been the cancer, it would have been something else. We've all got something. This is life. This is how it works."*

I need to trust that my kids will have the strength, the resources, the willingness, and the courage to deal with their own cancer fallout if and when they need to, just as Blondie is doing now.

*Tales from Clark Street (http://talesfromclarkstreet.blogspot.com)

▨ Monday, September 3, 2007

Uneven Terrain

Sometimes, my heart is so full of joy that I feel it might burst out of my chest. Sometimes, my heart is so heavy with sadness for everything I've lost that I can barely move. And sometimes, I feel both ways at the same time.

Just Another Mom in the Schoolyard

Sacha told me this weekend, as we were heading out for a dog walk, that I look "just like all the other moms." He sounded so happy when he said it, and he made me feel very happy and proud.

He and I both understood what it meant to say that. He went on to say that he's very "relieved" that I don't wear that "fake rubber breast" and that he likes the way I look. He's a very special kid.

Daniel

When we left for our walk, you carefully buckled Horsie into the stroller seat beside you.

You made me stop four times to tell me that Horsie was falling asleep. You fell asleep.

You awoke suddenly, and called out my name. I stopped and gently asked what you wanted. You said, "I'm ready to go now," and fell back asleep.

When you were really awake, we went for dog food, cat food, and chocolate milk at the "dog cafe." The young women who work there fell for your charms. There were lots of marshmallows in your chocolate milk.

You told me that Horsie was thirsty.

I said he could have some water.

You said that Horsie prefers chocolate milk.

I told you that chocolate milk would give Horsie a stomach-ache.

You said it would be okay because Horsie would have only a couple of sips. I asked you if you planned to drink the rest.

Horsie had to settle for water.

Did I mention that the young women who worked at the store fell for your charms?

You walked all the way home, proudly walking the dog all by yourself. It took us forty minutes to cover the fifteen-minute walk home. We had a big fight at the busiest intersection because I made you give me the leash and hold onto my hand.

Now it is after 10:00 and you are still awake.

You just came downstairs. I opened my mouth to scold you, but you said, "Mama, I can see the moon out my window. Come see."

We looked at the moon, I kissed you goodnight (yet again), and I tucked you in bed.

You look like me. You drive me to distraction. And I love you to distraction.

Happy, Happy, Happy

I saw my oncologist today. He examined me and decided that he does not need to see me for two whole months. This means that my weeks off will be genuinely "off" from the cancer centre. Even better, my lymph nodes all seem normal, my chest sounds clear, and he couldn't even feel the edge of my liver.

What a difference a year (or even less) can make.

The nurse was commenting on how heavy my cancer centre file is. I answered, "That's good. As long as it keeps getting heavier, it means that I'm still around."

■ **Thursday, September 13, 2007**

Badass Superhero

Yesterday, the Junky's Wife*, one of my online friends and an awesome woman in her own right, called me a "badass." This made my day. She also said that I should have my own superhero. Along with some of my other online friends, I have been having fun imagining what she would look like:

Super Me
a one-breasted warrior
with really great boots
a Rhea Belle** top
and some seriously funky accessories (thanks to Babz*** for that
suggestion)
generous hips (the better to shoot from)
crow's feet
and smile lines
honest
smart
strong
and always compassionate
but ready to kick ass
when she needs to.

* http://www.thejunkyswife.com

** designed by my friend Jacqueline, who creates clothes for the post-mastectomy body (http://rebel1in8.com/rhea.html)

*** http://lovebabz.blogspot.com

■ **Monday, September 17, 2007**

Sulking

I really don't want to go to chemo tomorrow. After two weeks off, I feel really good, and I'm too busy for chemo. Of course, I *will* go, but I don't have to be happy about it. I'll try to imagine the chemo zapping all the stray cancer cells tomorrow, and then the Herceptin getting anything the chemo misses. But tonight, I'm pissed off. I think I'm going to go pour myself a scotch.

Irreplaceable

On a recent train trip, my son lost his MP3 player. We had been on the way to Grandma's house and Sacha had much of his gear scattered around him. He had been quietly reading and working on the computer when he suddenly announced that he was not feeling well.

I won't inflict the gory details of what happened next upon my readers. Suffice it to say that my boy has not brought up so much over such an extended period of time since the Great Rosh Hashanah Puke-fest of 1999. It was grim, very grim.

When the dust had settled and once clothes were washed and boots were scrubbed, I realized that we had not made it off the train without leaving some things behind. While still on the train, I had put all of the still-clean contents of my son's backpack into a garbage bag, while putting the things that would need to be washed into another. Somehow my son's thumb drive and MP3 player did not make the transfer, or perhaps we lost them when the bag fell apart, clattering his belongings all over the floor of the train station. I can't be sure. At least these lost things are replaceable.

When Sacha was very young, he had a small stuffed dog. Little Dog (at that stage in his life, he named his toys very prosaically) went everywhere with him. Small enough to fit in the palm of my hand, we lived in fear of losing this toy to which my son was very deeply attached. Little Dog was lost and then recovered several times. We found him once in a tree outside my son's daycare, another time in the middle of an intersection in front of the airport. Then one day he was lost for good, having perhaps fallen out of a car on a day full of errands.

Six years later, my son still cannot bear to talk about it. I understand this. More than once, I have put dolls and stuffed animals on buses so that they could make their way home to children who have left them behind. And once, on vacation, my father sent a taxi back to a hotel some distance away to recover my beloved stuffed kangaroo. More than thirty years later, ratty old Skippy still resides in my bedroom closet.

But an MP3 player, I console myself, can be replaced.

And some day, I am sure I'll be ready to take the train with my son again.

Seven Random Facts about Me

1. I had my nose pierced when I was twenty-one. I was in India (on Canada World Youth) and a bunch of us had it done at the same time. The piercing was done with a sharpened piece of copper wire. That is how I found out that ...

2. I am allergic to copper.

3. I am the poster child for the programs of the post-Lester Pearson/Pierre Trudeau era in Canada. I participated in the Terry Fox Centre (a week-long session on government for sixteen-year-olds from across Canada); attended Lester B. Pearson College of the Pacific (200 students—fifty from Canada, the rest from all over the world—all of us on scholarship, in residence for two years, in Victoria, British Columbia); taught French to children of francophone parents (I worked in Powell River, BC); and participated in the aforementioned Canada World Youth. All great examples of Canadian tax dollars at work. Many of the things I have since achieved can be attributed to the foundation created by these programs.

4. I ran a half-marathon in October 2000. I trained and ran it with my sister, who willingly slowed herself to my pace. I will never forget her encouraging words as we climbed up that last hill (University Avenue, for those who know Toronto) and I whimpered that I wasn't going to make it: "You are damn

well going to finish this thing!" It is still one of my proudest achievements and I never could have done it without her.

5. I admit this guiltily, but I was relieved to give birth to two boys.

6. I hated being pregnant and suffered from antenatal depression, which lifted immediately after giving birth.

7. I am a compulsive list-maker. I keep lists of just about anything you can imagine.

Ongoing or Never-ending?

First Conversation

NURSE *(doing my pre-chemo blood-draw)*: "So are you almost done?"

ME: "No."

NURSE *(chirping)*: "Yup!"

ME: "I have metastatic cancer, so treatment will continue for the foreseeable future."

NURSE: "Yup!"

Second Conversation

NURSE *(setting up my chemo)*: "You must be almost done."

ME: "No, actually. I have metastatic cancer and will be in treatment for some time."

NURSE: "Well, they usually only give Herceptin for a year."

ME *(too worn out to explain that when Herceptin is being used to treat cancer that has spread or is metastatic, treatment can continue for years)*: "Hmmm."

Am I wrong to hold health care providers to a higher standard? Don't get me wrong. The nurses are, generally speaking, wonderful and busy, so I don't expect each one of them to have read my chart, but shouldn't oncology nurses know enough about differences in treatment protocols to not ask these kinds of questions if they don't really have an interest in the answers?

Just asking.

■ **Thursday, September 27, 2007**

"I HAVE CANCER AND I AM PISSED"

That's what someone Googled to find my blog today.

I love it. And whoever you are, I hope you found what you were looking for there.

Not in My Name

In 1992, when I adopted my first dog, I started noticing dogs everywhere I went.

When I was first pregnant and then became a mom, it seemed like every woman I saw was having a baby.

So last October, when it seemed to me that the whole world had turned pink, I first chalked this up to my own increased awareness. Then I realized that there was something much more insidious behind the pink-ribbon bandwagon, so I wrote about it a year ago in the post, entitled "Not Enough to Think Pink."

These are just some of the things I came across or was asked to promote in the lead-up to Breast Cancer Awareness Month, 2007:

- Pink acrylic sweaters with little pink ribbons on them

- Pink vacuum cleaners

- Pink towels promoting a sports beverage

- Pink candies

- Pink manicures (There is a nail place down the street from me that is decorated in pink that claims to donate part of its profits to "fight breast cancer." I mean, I love a good pedicure as much as the next girl, but do you know *how many carcinogens there are in nail polish?*)

- Pink coffee mugs

- Pink yogourt

- Pink soup

When someone you love gets cancer, it is very normal and understandable to feel that you want to do something for her, but please don't let that inclination lead you to buy some crappy, plastic doohickey that was made under dubious working conditions and that created carcinogenic by-products in the process.

Resist the urge to buy something pink just because the company tells you that some of the proceeds will go to "fight breast cancer" (fight it how, exactly?). If I sound pissed off, it's because I am. I resent big corporations, many of which have built empires contributing to rising cancer rates, increasing their profit margin while improving their philanthropic image. And I resent that this disease, which has ravaged my body, shortened my life, and cost me so much, is associated with the kind of pale-pink crap that idealizes a kind of subservient femininity that I loathe. I resent big businesses getting richer when breast cancer patients get poorer. And I really resent feeling exploited.

Suzanne Reisman* is a contributing editor at BlogHer, and she wrote the following in a recent post, "Pink Ribbon Madness: Say No to Breast Cancer Exploitation for Corporate Profit":

> Corporations push breast cancer in October because it works to sell more products. Women worry that some day they will face breast cancer or already know someone who has. They want to help. And what way is better than to buy something that promises to do good? The reality is that very little of the amount women spend on the pink products wind up at charitable institutions. An ABC News Report from last October pointed out that Campbell's

donated a whopping 3.5 cents for every can of soup it sold. To raise a mere $36 to fight breast cancer from the Yoplait campaign, a person needs to eat three cups of yogurt a day for four months.

Some companies may well be genuinely well-intentioned, and sometimes they donate all of the profits from a particular product to breast cancer research, but even this leaves a bad taste in my mouth.

Jeanne Sather**, who writes the blog *Assertive Cancer Patient*, explains this well in a post entitled "Gag me with a Pink Ribbon" (I love that title!):

> [In 2004] I work[ed] as a freelance Web writer for the Seattle Cancer Care Alliance, where I'm also a patient, receiving ongoing treatment for metastatic breast cancer. I recently sampled the pink dessert at the Dahlia Lounge in order to write about it for the SCCA site—and it was delicious.... I enjoyed every bite, except for the ribbon, which I left on the side of my plate. The dessert costs $8. So let's do the math. You order the dessert for $8, plus a cup of coffee for, say, $2. Add in tax and tip, and the bill comes to about $13. Of that, the restaurant gives Athena [the non-profit benefiting from the donation] the net profit, generally between $3 and $4.... The Dahlia Lounge had sold thirty-four desserts in five days. So, say they sell 204 in the month; that's only a donation of about $800. Pocket change. One small research project costs hundreds of thousands of dollars a year, if not more.
>
> There's a simpler solution: Skip dessert and send $8, or the whole $13, directly to your favorite hospital or research center.

If you really, really want that piece of cake with pink frosting, by all means, go ahead and indulge. Just don't do it in my name, okay?

* BlogHer (http://www.blogher.com) and Campaign for Unshaved Snatch (CUSS) & Other Rants (http://cussandotherrants.com)

** http://www.assertivepatient.com

Etching Myself in Their Memories

"I'm starting to forget Emma."

Sacha said this to me a couple of days ago. Our old dog died last summer. She was very nearly fourteen and had had a great life, but her passing was a sad event for my little family.

"I can't really remember what she looked like or the things she liked to do," he went on.

"That's perfectly normal," I replied.

"Is it?"

"Yes, and that's why we tell stories about our loved ones who've died, to help each other remember them."

"Like the time Emma almost drowned Grandpa?"

"That's right, and you have lots of pictures, too."

That was pretty much the end of our conversation, but it did put a lump in my throat. I may be in remission, but I do know what the statistics are when it comes to stage 4 breast cancer. I try not to torture myself with these, but I know that I will likely die long before I am ready. The thought that I might become a hazy memory to my children is something else on which I try not to dwell, but it hurts.

This morning, I was cuddling with my youngest, covering his little head with kisses. I felt both intensely happy and very, very sad.

"Remember this moment," I wanted to whisper. "Remember me."

Making Like a Duck

It wasn't supposed to be like this.

My spouse is away on a well-deserved vacation and I am playing at being a single parent. I had been imagining all the fun things my kids and I would do together—go for bike rides, to the park, the library. I would get my writing and errands out of the way today and even have time for lunch with a friend I haven't seen for a couple of years.

But the weather sucks, my oldest has been testing his limits, and my four-year-old has come down with a miserable cold. I cancelled my lunch date, am behind on my writing, and feeling like the world's worst mother (how many consecutive hours should any child be allowed to watch TV, even when he's sick?).

My spouse left yesterday, so Daniel and I put on a CD this morning and danced around. I promised Sacha a movie this evening. Things may not be going the way that I'd planned, but we'll roll with it.

The minute that the sun comes out, I am throwing on some clothes (did I mention that I am still in my pyjamas?), bundling Daniel in the stroller and going for a walk. I'm washing my hands a lot so that I don't get sick. I'll see if I can set up a play date for Sacha this weekend. In the days before cancer, this turn of events would have left me feeling pretty bitter. Now I'm only a little bitter.

Enough for Today

I have been struggling a little these last few weeks. It was around this time last year and the year before that cancer changed my life. I've been finding it hard to shake the grief and anxiety. But today, I experienced a moment that quite literally took my breath away. I was out walking my dog in the arboretum, pretty much lost in thought, when I was taken off guard by a tree, a pond, the sunset, and scattered leaves in all my favourite colours. And the thought suddenly came to me: I am grateful.

Grateful for my kids for bringing me joy, making me laugh, and for needing me. Grateful for my spouse, who is kind and gentle and who loves me even when I am crazy. Grateful for my dog who gets me out walking. Grateful for a lovely walk in a beautiful place. And grateful that I am healthy and fit enough to enjoy it all. Tomorrow remains uncertain, but for today, it is enough to be grateful.

Lap Cat Distracts from CAT Scan Worries (Dog Snoring Does a Pretty Good Job Too)

I am exhausted. I have to get up early tomorrow to go to for abdominal and thoracic CT scans (also known as CAT scans).

Once someone has had cancer, every headache, stitch, lump, bump, or bout of dizziness becomes suspect. And every test, no matter how routine, is fraught with anxiety.

I have been the best kind of busy these last few days. I've just returned from the National Conference for Young Women Living with Breast Cancer. The time spent with friends and family while I was there, as well as the chance to change my environment for a while, provided both a distraction and more reassurance than a fist full of tranquilizers.

But I do feel a little queasy and a lot scared when I think about what the results of this test could mean. The worst doesn't bear thinking about, actually, so I'm trying not to do so. And right now, with my youngest asleep, my oldest in the bath, my sweetie in the room with me, the dog snoring with his head in my lap, and the cat doing his best imitation of a nice kitty, it's not so hard to feel optimistic. I just wish the test was over, the results were in, and that I could share the good news with all of you.

I Am Spectacular

The results are in:

My liver functions are normal. The condition of my liver has improved. There is no evidence at all of metastasis—no sign that I have cancer at all, in fact. Why am I so surprised by this? I have had a dull ache (sometimes a sharper pain) in the area of my liver for the last couple of weeks. It's exactly where the stitch started last year, the stitch that led to the discovery that my cancer had spread. I have had moments of pure unadulterated terror when I have thought about what it could mean.

It turns out that the pain, which I had been hoping was in my head (but knew in my heart to be real), is due to scarring. You know how scar tissue is so tight and inflexible? The scars on my liver are causing it to retract, making it sensitive.

My oncologist seemed even happier than he was back in July when we first discovered my tumours had disappeared. "It's all gone!" he crowed.

I was relieved and overjoyed, but felt the need to reassure him that I was also being realistic about my prognosis. The longer we can maintain the status quo, the better, but I do know that one day this treatment will stop working.

But he surprised me. He said, "Well, realistic.... For some women the results of combining Herceptin and Vinorelbine have been spectacular."

Spectacular.

And then he added, "I think you might continue this way for a long, long time." He concluded by telling my friend Theresa to take me out for a drink, which she did.

"Go celebrate."

I did have a glass of wine. Now I am going to put my four-year-old to bed and then collapse out of sheer exhaustion and relief.

And tomorrow? I am going to go back to being spectacular.

Not Waiting for the Other Shoe

The night after my CT, I dreamed that my dog Jasper had been in a terrible accident. In the dream, I rushed to the hospital and waited, feeling anxious, terrified, and grief-stricken while he was in surgery. In the end, my dear dog survived the accident and was expected to recover. He was, however, really traumatized. It wasn't until I was recounting this dream at the breakfast table that I realized that it hadn't been about the dog at all.

Back in July, when I got the first good CT result, I was overjoyed at first, but then angst-ridden. And the reality is that while I have now twice received the best news possible, my day-to-day life will not change very much. I will continue with chemo—two weeks on, two weeks off. I am still a cancer patient.

But as I continue to defy the odds (the stats on survival rates for women with metastatic breast cancer are abysmal and the stats when the metastasis is in the liver are even worse), I need to give myself permission to let down my guard a little—to be hopeful.

It's starting to feel okay to make plans for a few months in the future, and in a few months, perhaps I will feel I can plan even further ahead than that.

My friend Theresa said to me as we left my appointment on Tuesday, "You are going to get to see your kids grow up." I am not sure I'm ready to let myself believe that, but I replay her words to myself and I feel warmed by them.

I'm starting with teaching myself not to panic whenever I feel the familiar stitch in my side. I know now that the pain is due to scarring, but I am still working on quieting the panic it instills, so not much has changed, but everything has changed.

I can't have my old life back, but I have a great deal of hope. I think I can live with that.

On Life as a Pincushion

I am covered in some spectacular bruises. To do the CT, they not only have to find a vein, they have to thread the needle through it in order to create an IV for radioactive dye. If this sounds painful, it's because it is, and veins on someone who's had a lot of chemo are hard to come by.

First, they tried on the inside of my elbow. Then they tried on the side of my forearm. Finally, they had to go for the inside of my wrist. The nurse informed me that she usually avoids this at all costs because it is "torture." She actually said this more than once. It hurt like hell. I think the nurse was astonished that I didn't yell or lose my temper. I did gasp, and rather loudly, as the murmurs from those waiting on the other side of the curtain indicated. But I was good (as we first-born children tend to be).

The nurse kept commenting on how good-natured I was. I'm certainly more stoic than I used to be, but really, though, I was too stressed about getting the test done to think much about being stuck with needles.

It's all relative, really.

■ Monday, November 19, 2007

All the Experts

Recently, someone who ought to know better, a professional to whom I had turned for tools to deal with fear and anxiety, said to me, "People who spend their lives saying that everything is a pain in the neck often find that that is where they get cancer."

My eyes widened. My tone sharpened. I asked, "Are you telling me that I got breast cancer because I had negative feelings about my body?"

"Well, I am not talking about blame here, but many people who grow up hearing negative things or thinking negatively about a particular body part end up, years later, getting cancer in exactly that part of their body."

Excuse me? What young woman doesn't grow up thinking at least somewhat negatively about her body, especially one who goes through puberty as young as I did? And, yeah, I did hear lots of negative comments about my body when I was young. And, yes, I have hated both my breasts and my belly at times.

But I repeat: What woman doesn't feel at least some ambivalence about her body?

He kept saying that he got this idea from Bernie Siegel in *Love, Medicine, and Miracles*. I haven't read that book, but I did read another by him (*Peace, Love, and Healing*), and I suspect that his words were distorted by this so-called therapist.

The whole session with this man was appalling. He rambled, said a number of inappropriate and irrelevant things about himself and other clients, and seemed to have little inclination to listen to what

I was saying (and I ended up saying very little). He was extremely irritated when I ended the session early. I stayed for an hour, but really, I was ready to bolt after the first five minutes.

I left feeling more than a little shaken and relieved that I had not gone to see this fraud when I was actually feeling vulnerable like, say, right after I had learned of the metastasis. The good news I have just received has helped me to feel healthy and strong. Still, this guy managerd to seriously unsettle me.

When it comes to cancer, there are many folks who purport to have all the answers. You don't have to go too far outside the mainstream to find self-styled experts who claim to know what causes cancer and how to cure it. Of course, any failings on their part are blamed on the patients themselves.

This is why I stopped going to my acupuncturist, other than the fact that he was acutely paranoid and that I once found a needle still stuck in my belly after I got home. One day, I overheard the woman in the next bed (we were separated only by a curtain) tell the good "doctor" that her cancer had returned. "It's because you stopped coming to me," he told her. And then, "Chemotherapy doesn't work." The woman actually agreed and apologized to him. I didn't say anything, but I left that day and never went back. I know that acupuncture really does help with chemo's side effects, but for me, the stress and the pain of the visits weren't worth it.

And although my naturopathic doctor is a lovely woman, I found myself leaving each appointment laden with more supplements. And for a while, I was injecting myself with Iscador, a mistletoe derivative that is commonly prescribed in Germany, but not covered by Canadian insurance. My ND did produce studies to back up her claims that Iscador is a wonder drug, but in the end, that too proved overwhelming. I just couldn't bring myself to keep spending money on something in which I didn't fully believe. I already have to inject myself with Neupogen (to keep my white blood counts up) ten times a month. I really have had enough of needles.

The bottom line is that I trust my oncologist, and the treatment he has prescribed for me seems to be working. Even if there are alternatives out there that could work just as well or even better, I have to choose to put my faith somewhere.

I also need to figure out who and what can help complement my cancer treatment to help me feel strong and fit and healthy. Navigating the various claims and contradictions is a little overwhelming right at the moment, and I am feeling a bit burned by the incompetent therapist, so I think I'll give myself a little time off from the "experts."

Serendipity

Sometimes the most amazing things happen, or are done by amazing people.

Two weeks ago we had nineteen people at our house for a family Chanukah party. The cooking was shared (my spouse refers to Chanukah as "the festival of fried things"), the cleanup was shared, and everyone had a great time.

After the meal, the children in the family exchanged presents. There was also a package with my name on it. As I started to protest that this was against the rules, I was told that it was something special from my oldest niece, who will be twelve this year.

It turned out that she had knit me a hat. It was her first non-scarf project and it is perfect. It's the most beautiful shade of turquoise, fits beautifully, and just happens to be the exact same colour as the turquoise flecks in the scarf that I wear every day. And it looks great on me. Just that week, I had tried to knit myself a hat, but there was something wrong with my yarn or the pattern and it hadn't worked out. Just that day, I had been thinking how much I love it when people knit things for me and that I wish it would happen more often.

I love that hat with a passion because it is perfect and because it was so thoughtfully and carefully made, just for me.

And I have another example of an amazing thing. I have been feeling kind of down lately—part Chanukah letdown, part grief for my old life, and part chemotherapy blues. I've been feeling the dogs of depression nipping at my ankles. I've been fighting them off, and figuring out how to be healthier, but it has been a bit of a struggle and, of course, the sadness is compounded by the guilt of a recovering Catholic: "I should be ashamed to be feeling so sorry for myself when I have responded to treatment so well, have good insurance, and such great support!"

Two days ago, I wrote about feeling uninspired. Yesterday, a beautiful knitting book appeared in my mailbox, bound with a ribbon, on which was written the following: "I like reading your blog and I find inspiration from it. Here is a book for you, may it bring you inspiration."

It was from Julie, an artist friend, with whom I once worked closely and haven't seen in a long time. To think I inspire her means a great deal to me.

You know the expression "my heart lifted"? I now know exactly how that feels. And how could she possibly have known that I have been scouring the Internet for patterns for knitted bags?

Sometimes, life is very hard. And it's not true that everything happens for a reason. But sometimes, the right thing happens at exactly the right time, or good people know how to make good things happen.

Thursday, January 3, 2008

Where Inspiration Comes from

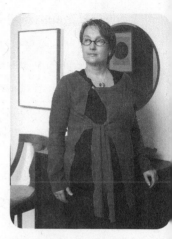

Last December, I flew to New York City to stay with my friend Jacqueline, a very talented artist, a cancer survivor, and the designer of Rhea Belle Apparel for the post-mastectomy body.

I approached this trip with excitement, but also a fair amount of trepidation. Jacqueline and I had never met in person or even spoken on the phone. I had never been to New York City, and it had been a long time since I had travelled by myself to any new place, but I was ready for adventure and highly motivated.

I don't use the term "kindred spirits" easily, but I felt a connection to Jacqueline from the moment we met on the pavement in front of her house. This was preceded by a moment of panic when the taxi dropped me off outside a building that looked decidedly non-residential, in the middle of what seemed like industrial wasteland. It was all illusion—the former factory housed breathtaking artists' lofts. We started to talk as the elevator made its way up to Jacqueline's floor and were still talking when John, Jacqueline's husband, joined us a few hours later. The three of us remained at their kitchen table until long after my bedtime.

I did have many adventures that weekend, some with Jacqueline (loved that Brooklyn pizza!) and some by myself. I walked for hours in Manhattan, making my way from Battery Park to the Chelsea Hotel (historic home to many great writers), past Macy's Christmas window, through the garment district (where I could have bought a North Face coat for a couple of bucks), to the New York Public Library (where I spent hours; admission is free and it's an amazing place), and on to Times Square.

I had tons of energy and felt confident, even among the crowds. Jacqueline and John may have been humouring me, but they complimented me hugely when they said that I looked like a New Yorker, not like a tourist. It felt great.

On my last evening, we discussed a visit I had made that day to the Guggenheim. Jacqueline and John shared some of their own art with me, along with the thoughts that had gone into the process of making it. I talked a bit about writing and reflected that I was trying to think of myself as a creative person.

The look on John's face at that moment was a gift. He was incredulous. I can't remember exactly what he said, but he told me that if I can write a blog or a book, then I am a writer. And if I am a writer, then I am creative.

I have thought of that moment many times in the weeks since my trip.

Jacqueline tells me that she sometimes feels criticized by other artists because she designs clothing now instead of making more traditional art, but every item of clothing and jewellery she makes is imbued with her passion and shaped by her talent. I feel beautiful, strong, and powerful when I adorn my asymmetrical body with her creations.

My visit to New York inspired me in ways that go beyond the clothing I brought home and the places I visited. I returned with a new sense of myself as a creative person, an artist in my own right, who uses words to paint pictures of the world around me.

■ Thursday, January 10, 2008

Reports of My (Imminent) Death Are Greatly Exaggerated

I have this book with a flowchart in it. It shows how cancer cells mutate and grow. It has lots of little arrows pointing to the possibilities. Cancerous cells can be treated and eradicated, or turn into a cancerous tumour. A tumour can be zapped with chemo and disappear, or it can metastasize. Once cancer is beaten, a person may be "recovered," or they may have a "recurrence." But there is only one arrow leading from "metastases," and it points toward "death." This flowchart really upset me when I saw it (it's in a freakin' cookbook!) and it pissed me off.

Then I went to the National Conference for Young Women Living with Breast Cancer. There were only a handful of us there with metastastic breast cancer (six or seven out of a few hundred, I'd say), but one was a conference organizer, and we all looked pretty damn good. More of us are getting breast cancer, and we're getting it at younger ages, but we are also living longer, and living well.

My oncologist and I talked about this yesterday. As I have said before, I've had "spectacular" results with my current treatment regimen. Figuring out next steps, though, is a bit of a guessing game. The following is from breastcancer.org:

> Many women can live for years with metastatic cancer that's under control. For these women, living with a diagnosis of metastatic breast cancer is like living with a chronic disease. It can go into remission, be active sometimes and not others, or move quickly. It frequently involves trying one treatment after another, ideally

with breaks in-between treatments when you feel good. The goal of treatment is to help you feel as well as possible and live a longer life.

No one can tell you how long you will live with metastatic disease. That's because every woman's experience is different. Some women live for more than a decade. Others live for just a few seasons. But new and more effective treatments keep being developed. This means that you may do much better today with metastatic disease than someone who had it only a few years ago.

In this phase of breast cancer, the treatment goal is to extend life as long as possible with the best QUALITY of life possible. This means relieving symptoms and putting cancer into remission with the fewest side effects.

I have already gone from a three-week cycle (with one week off from treatment) to a four-week cycle (with two weeks off from treatment). Now my doctor and I are discussing moving to a cycle where I would receive only one treatment every four weeks.

I have a lot of faith in my oncologist, who says that many women have had success on this kind of cycle, but that we have no way of knowing exactly the right amount of chemo needed to keep my cancer at bay. We also don't really know the long-term effects of Herceptin, which can potentially be damaging to the heart, because the drug is just too new.

The side effects of the drugs I'm on are relatively mild, but I am feeling emotionally and physically ground down by ongoing treatment. Chemotherapy attacks the healthy cells as well as the cancerous ones, and my body and soul have been paying the price. My heart leapt at the suggestion that I might get more of a break in the near future.

There are no easy answers, but the questions I have to ask are a whole lot more pleasant than ones I thought I might be facing a year ago, and I'm a damned sight better off than I would have been had all this happened to me even five years ago. I do know this, however: Metastasis may lead to death (we are all, after all, going to face death at some point), but until then, I plan to live fully and well.

Pavlov Revisited

One morning, as I was making school lunches, I dropped a piece of cheese on my dog's head. I had been slicing it onto sandwiches and had turned to talk to my older son. Multitasking before sufficient caffeine intake has never been my strong suit.

Now, whenever I am making lunches, the dog dances with excitement, his eyes sparkling with hope and joyful anticipation.

I want to live my life like that. Life is good, and you never know when cheese might fall from the sky.

Conclusion

AS I WRITE THIS, in late spring of 2008, I have had four clean CT scans. There continues to be no sign of cancer on my liver, just the scarring that remains as evidence of the once "innumerable" tumours. I have lost count of the number of chemotherapy and Herceptin treatments I have undergone.

I worry at times about the long-term effects of this kind of treatment. Herceptin can be damaging to the heart, so I continue to go for regular heart scans. I also worry about the carcinogenic potential of all these scans and injections with radioactive dye. My oncologist admits that we are charting new territory with my treatment. Even ten years ago, these options would not have been open to me, and if

I had been diagnosed ten years earlier, my prognosis would be much gloomier, so I am more than willing to be a bit of a guinea pig.

I will always be a cancer patient. When someone asks, "When will you stop treatment?" I always answer, "When it stops working." And then we will move on to something else. For now, though, I am thrilled with how well I have responded to treatment (so well that my oncologist has suggested I phone in for most of my appointments with him) and I remind myself of this when the grind starts to get me down.

All in all, I live a very good life and I feel healthy and strong most of the time. This has become my message, a refrain I repeat constantly for myself and others: "More of us are living well and longer than ever before." We are the new face of stage 4, or "metastatic" breast cancer, as it becomes, for us, a chronic illness that must be managed, but does not stop us from active participation in the world.

I still struggle at times with the ways in which cancer has irrevocably changed my life. I miss working. I still miss my right breast, and I resent the side effects of treatment as well as the scars from surgery and radiation, the lymphedema, the loss of range of motion in my right arm, and the ramifications of being post-menopausal at forty years old. But mostly, I am happy to be alive, and I am proud of myself.

Having cancer has taught me how strong I am and how lucky. It has also given me an awareness of my own abilities and put me back in touch with my creative spirit. Metastatic cancer has not ended my life; it has just caused me to live my life differently.

Looking back on the last year, my trips to New York and to Chicago marked real turning points. I was reminded that the world is still full of interesting things to do, experience, and write about. I learned that being creative is about taking risks and having eyes that are open and a spirit that is receptive. I began to think of myself as an artist and writer.

I now write almost every day. I take long walks with my dog and volunteer at my son's school. (I'm teaching the kids in his grade 4 class how to knit.) I am working on taking better care of myself and treating myself with more compassion.

I am learning to live in the moment.

I have begun to plan, tentatively, for the future.

In some ways I feel that cancer has made me into more well-rounded person. I am a cancer patient, but also a mother, spouse, friend, sister, activist, writer, and many other things I have yet to discover.

I would never choose to have cancer. I still don't believe that "cancer is a gift," but my life with cancer is infinitely better than I would ever have thought possible.

Acknowledgments

I COULD FILL ANOTHER BOOK with the names of people who have helped me survive and grow during the last couple of years. I want to especially thank the following folks who, in various ways, helped make this book become a reality:

First of all, Susan, Jack, and Women's Press for proposing this project and making me believe I could do it. And thank you, too, for your overwhelming support and generosity in more ways that I can count.

My mom, for loving unconditionally, being the first person to make me laugh, and for being chauffeur, stage mom, costume designer, and advocate. You made so many happy memories possible.

My father, for teaching me to love language and writing, for encouraging me to work hard at both, and for taking so much pride in my successes.

My beautiful, talented sister for being my first fan and continuing to be my most valued critic.

My editor, Rebecca Conolly, for being so good at it.

My chemo posse, for making the hardest part of my life seem like so much fun.

My friends and co-workers who sent me to BlogHer in Chicago in 2007. You gave me something to anticipate when I needed it most and helped create memories that have carried me through the hard times.

PSAC, for being the kind of employer every cancer patient should have.

Deb, Leslie, Andrea, and Helen.

Every friend who has stood by me and expressed your support in so many ways. Thank you for every meal, gift, message, joke, phone call, blog comment, hug, and Scrabble game, and thank you especially for making me feel so loved.

My community of online friends. You have come to mean so much to me, across distance and difference. Our commonalities bring us together, and I know I am never alone.

Joyce Hardman, for giving the best advice ever and without whom I would have spent a lot more time whimpering under my desk.

My Six Sisters of the Dragon, for all that we share and what we create together.

Ian H., Ian W., Dawn, Zoe, Emma, Andrew, Brenda, Claire, Esmé, Noah, Sarah, Adam, Nate, Corinne, and especially Susan. I am so fortunate to have each of you in my family.

Bonnie, for the BlogHer idea, for the chart for recruiting and organizing volunteers, but mostly for being so formidable.

Liam for letting the head shaving be a performance.

GB for "lucky," "borrowed time," and so many other reasons.

My amazing boys, for providing distraction, inspiration, and motivation, and for being the reason I get up every morning.

And, above all, Tim—my love, sounding board, cheerleader, co-conspirator, foundation, and soul mate. I love you more than I can say.